I0093180

Shut Up & Die

By

Harold Godspeed

Copyright © 2023 Harold Godspeed

All rights reserved.

ISBN: 979-8-218-25458-2

DISCLAIMER

This book and its contents do not cure, prevent, diagnose or treat any disease or condition. The information, facts and opinions presented are for entertainment and not intended as a substitute for the advice, diagnosis or treatment of a licensed medical professional. This information is not medical advice or opinion; in no way should anyone infer that the author is practicing medicine by the information and opinions provided.

If you have an illness, disease or life-threatening emergency, please contact a doctor or go to a hospital. This publication represents the author's opinions, which are based on his beliefs, knowledge and experiences. The techniques, theories and regimens in this book are not prescriptions or recommendations. The techniques, theories and regimens listed in this publication do not represent a scientific consensus, prevention or self-help. You agree to use all information, techniques, regimens and information published in this book at your own risk, based upon your own free will. Before starting any new program, supplementation, diet, technique or regimen, please consult your physician or integrative medicine specialist, especially if you have a specific illness, condition or disease or are taking any medication.

This book is for education, entertainment and research. Be advised that the entire content of this publication is solely the opinion of the author and do not represent any of the cited materials, persons or ideas in this book.

The publisher, author and any cited materials or persons in this book take no responsibility for the outcomes or results of any of the information in this book.

If you think you have or may have a health condition described in this book DO NOT ATTEMPT any of the ideas, techniques, regimens, knowledge or comments in this book without consulting a competent health care professional first.

Before we begin...

Many of the statements about companies, manufacturing processes or intentions of use, intentions of the company or implied nefarious nature of any said entity are opinion and speculation and are for informational and educational purposes.

The author, publisher and everyone involved directly or indirectly with the publication, distribution and sale of this book assume no responsibility for any outcome the reader may encounter.

The author, publisher or any other involved parties do not assume liability for the use or misuse of any of the information contained herein, be it direct or indirect, mental, physical, consequential, special, exemplary or any other damages. The aforementioned do not assume responsibility or liability for any complication from any information usage.

All rights reserved. No part of this book may be used or reproduced in any manner whatsoever or stored in any database or retrieval system without written permission except in the case of brief quotations used in critical articles and reviews.

The scanning, uploading and distribution of this book without permission is theft of the author's intellectual property. If you would like permission to use material from this book other than for review purposes, please contact *shutupanddiebook@proton.me*.

TABLE OF CONTENTS

INTRODUCTION

We don't want you to die in the state you are in. Are you or a loved one plagued by continuing and increasing health problems? Maybe it is as mild as chronic fatigue or maybe it has morphed into multiple autoimmune issues. Maybe it has even progressed to cancer or mental health issues that have changed your lifestyle and put you in fear of death. Whatever it is, it is becoming a bigger and bigger issue to the point that it may feel insurmountable.

We want you to live—not just continue on in the state you are in but live a vibrant healthy life again—spiritually, physically and mentally. And there are answers to what is plaguing you!

By reading this book, you will be introduced not only to the root causes of all of these problems but also how you can find the answers you need to address the specifics of what is ailing you in your multifaceted being of soul, body and mind. This book will provide you with the tools and foundations to not only research what has caused your illness but how to find answers to help you recover a healthier lifestyle.

PART ONE:

SAVE YOUR SOUL

- 1 -

THE FEAR OF THE LORD IS THE BEGINNING OF WISDOM

What is the foundation of your life? To do anything well, you must have a good foundation to build on—it filters your worldview and how you see everything. There are only two foundations and two "religions" in the world.

1) Those who build their foundation on the Rock (Christ) and obtain eternal salvation by grace *or*

2) Those who try to succeed by works righteousness (all other religions) and doing things their own way.

You must begin your journey into truth with this simple message, "the fear of the LORD is the beginning of wisdom" (Proverbs 9:10).

Let us begin to be wise with this simple exercise. There is a heaven and a hell and as soon as you die, you pass instantly from the temporal world into eternity and you must stand before God and give an account of your deeds.

Will you pass the test?

If you measure yourself against God's standard, you will know how you will stand on that day of accounting. By looking at the Ten Commandments in Exodus 20:3-17, you can judge for yourself whether you will be held guilty or not guilty according to God.

1. You shall have no other gods before Me.
2. You shall worship no idols.
3. You shall not take the name of the Lord your God in vain.

4. Keep the Sabbath day holy.
5. Honor your father and your mother.
6. You shall not murder.
7. You shall not commit adultery.
8. You shall not steal.
9. You shall not bear false witness against your neighbor.
10. You shall not covet.

As we go through a few of the commandments, examine yourself against them. Take note of how many of God's laws you have broken and this will give you a clear answer on where you will stand before God at judgment. I am not judging you; this is for you to examine yourself and see your current condition. You will not accept the cure if you do not know you have the disease.

ARE YOU SPIRITUALLY SICK?

You shall not take the name of the Lord your God in vain.

Have you ever used the name of God or Jesus as a swear word or not given it due honor? This is called blasphemy and it was a capital offense in Old Testament times.

You shall not murder.

Jesus said, "Everyone who hates his brother or sister is a murderer, and you know that no murderer has eternal life remaining in him." (1 John 3:15) Just hating someone makes you guilty of murder and if you could get away with it, you would probably do it.

You shall not commit adultery.

Jesus said, "You have heard that it was said, 'You shall not commit adultery'; but I say to you that everyone who looks at a woman with lust for her has already committed adultery with her in his heart." (Matthew 5:27-28) Have you ever lusted sexually after someone or watched pornography?

4

You shall not steal.

Have you ever stolen anything, regardless of the value? Even misrepresenting your time at work or using supplies from your job without reporting it is stealing.

You shall not bear false witness against your neighbor.

How many lies have you told? Have you been complicit in deceiving someone for your benefit? Lying can be by commission or omission.

You shall not covet.

Have you ever wanted, lusted after or plotted after something that is not yours? Have you been jealous because someone else got something you think you deserve more or they deserve less?

Examine yourself.

Stop and think for a moment on how God would judge these things from the standing of being perfectly holy and never having sinned at all.

THE SPIRITUAL CURE

Now that you have had a chance to read through the commandments and examine yourself against them, we can see how serious God is about us violating His law. Scripture says, "the soul that sins shall die" (Ezekiel 18:20) and "as it is appointed for men to die once, but after this the judgment" (Hebrews 9:27). "[T]he wages of sin is death" and so your death will be the evidence of the seriousness of God's wrath on sinners—your sins have separated you from God.

All of this is meant to put a little "fear of the Lord" in you so you can see the seriousness of your unsaved condition and how you will fare when you stand before the Lord at judgment. You will be guilty and condemned to an eternity in hell, a place of weeping, gnashing of teeth and eternal separation from God (Matthew 13:42).

So, what can you do to save yourself? Nothing! You cannot bribe God with your good works and no matter how many times you say you are sorry or that you will try harder, you will be without excuse.

The only thing you can do is humble yourself and throw yourself on the mercy of God. God *has* provided a way that you can be saved from the wrath to come—He sent His only Son as a living sacrifice on behalf of all who will believe (John 3:16). Jesus was crucified on the cross, died and was raised again on the third day. What happened on the cross is that Jesus paid the penalty for your sin— His death for yours. If you believe this and live in faith by it, when you stand before God, He will treat you as if you lived Jesus's life— perfect, sinless and holy—and He punished Christ for the sins you committed. On the cross, Jesus suffered separation from God and the torrent of God's wrath and when it was over, Christ said, "it is finished!" because the debt has been paid. Jesus conquered death and removed the sting of death for the believer—now, the believer walks through the shadow of death but will walk into a glorious eternity.

If you are reading this, please do not hesitate any longer, for you do not know the hour of your death and each moment you do not accept God's free gift, you are storing up wrath. Jesus said you "must be born again" (John 3:5-7). This is a greater miracle than your original birth—to be born again, you must acknowledge your sins, humble yourself before God, confess your sins to Him, repent or turn from those sins and trust in Christ for everything. When you do, you will be born again and God will give you a personal miracle and change you into a new creation (2 Corinthians 5:17). As a Christian, you will love righteousness and hate evil. The passage from earlier, "the wages of sin is death", continues with "but the gift of God is eternal life in Christ Jesus our Lord" (Romans 6:23). All you have to do is accept the gift—the free gift that you cannot earn or buy.

We can see a better illustration of this lesson by looking at the words of Jesus in Mark 10:17-22:

> As He was setting out on a journey, a man ran up to Him and knelt before Him, and asked Him, "Good Teacher, what shall I do so that I may inherit eternal life?" But Jesus said to him, "Why do you call Me good? No one is good except God alone. You know the commandments: 'Do not murder, Do not commit adultery, Do not steal, Do not give false testimony, Do not defraud, Honor your father and mother.'" And he said to Him, "Teacher, I have kept all these things from my youth." Looking at him, Jesus showed love to him and said to him, "One thing you lack: go and sell all you possess and give to the poor, and you will have treasure in heaven; and come, follow Me." But he was deeply dismayed by these words, and he went away grieving; for he was one who owned much property.

In this lesson, we see Jesus ask this young man about a few specific commandments, undoubtably knowing this young man's heart and true intentions. The man replied that he had kept all these commandments, but scripture tells the truth with these words "If we say that we have no sin, we deceive ourselves, and the truth is not in us. If we confess our sins, he is faithful and just to forgive us our sins, and to cleanse us from all unrighteousness. If we say that we have not sinned, we make him a liar, and his word is not in us." (1 John 1:8-10)

The young man may not have been outwardly sinful, but Jesus knew his heart and the true intentions of his actions. Jesus then asked the young man to sell off his possessions and follow Him. Jesus was not advocating for some system of communism or to not have possessions, but rather He was exposing this man's heart intentions and desires. The young man would rather serve his wealth and his sin than to forsake worldly pleasures and join Christ. In Mark 8:36, Jesus said, "For what shall it profit a man, if he shall gain the whole world, and lose his own soul?" And in Luke 9:23 "…He said to them all, if any man will come after me, let him deny himself, and take up his cross daily, and follow Me."

Sin may be pleasurable for a season, but it ends in death. Please examine my motivation—what do I gain for telling you this truth? It is my sincere prayer that you would be saved so I am speaking these things with truth in love to you for the sake of your soul.

Please recognize the exigent circumstances that you are in if you have not been forgiven and reconciled with God, "we are but a vapor" (James 4:14). You do not know when you will die so please take a moment, wherever you are at this moment, to humble yourself, cry out to the Lord for forgiveness, confess your sin before Him, turn away from your sin (repent) and believe that Christ has paid for your sin, that He was raised on the third day and then put your full trust in Christ. In a world that is rapidly deteriorating, you can have peace and hope in the life to come and you can tell others the Good News so that they may be saved also.

Please read the book of John in the Bible and visit the appendices for references and to explore the many resources that are listed there. Additionally, if you have any questions, please feel free to email *shutupanddiebook@proton.me* or to reach out to any of the spiritual resources listed at the end of this book.

A NEW OUTLOOK

Biblical Christianity is the lens through which you must view the world to have an understating of why things are the way they are and why they are so rapidly deteriorating—with your health, our society and the world in general. Sin is the reason why things are bad—sin entered the world and all of creation has been corrupted so now Satan is the "prince" of this world. (Ephesians 2:2)

RUN THROUGH ROMANS

Now that we have touched on the most important aspect of spirituality, we can examine why western civilization is collapsing and is under the judgement of God—why we have been abandoned by Him to the rapidly-progressing evil in our government and society. This section of scripture outlines the progression of all cultures when they abandon God. Romans 1:18-32 says:

> For the wrath of God is revealed from heaven against all ungodliness and unrighteousness of people who suppress the truth in unrighteousness, because that which is known about God is evident within them; for God made it evident to them. For since the creation of the world His invisible attributes, that is, His eternal power and divine nature, have been clearly perceived, being understood by what has been made, so that they are without excuse. For even though they knew God, they did not honor Him as God or give thanks, but they became futile in their reasonings, and their senseless hearts were darkened. Claiming to be wise, they became fools, and they exchanged the glory of the incorruptible God for an image in the form of corruptible mankind, of birds, four-footed animals, and crawling creatures.
>
> Therefore God gave them up to vile impurity in the lusts of their hearts, so that their bodies would be dishonored among them. For they exchanged the truth of God for falsehood, and worshiped and served the creature rather than the Creator, who is blessed forever. Amen. For this reason God gave them over to degrading passions; for their women exchanged natural relations for that which is contrary to nature, and likewise the men, too, abandoned natural relations with women and burned in their desire toward one another, males with males committing shameful acts and receiving in their own persons the due penalty of their error.
>
> And just as they did not see fit to acknowledge God, God gave them up to a depraved mind, to do those things that are not proper, people having been filled with all unrighteousness, wickedness, greed, and evil; full of envy, murder, strife, deceit, and malice; they are gossips, slanderers, haters of God, insolent, arrogant, boastful, inventors of evil, disobedient to parents, without understanding, untrustworthy, unfeeling, and unmerciful; and although they know the ordinance of God, that those who practice such things are worthy of death, they not only do the same, but also approve of those who practice them.

If we start with verse 18, *"For the wrath of God is revealed from heaven against all ungodliness and unrighteousness of people who suppress the truth in unrighteousness,"* we see this is clearly evident in our society as there is an all-out war on the truth and "Woe to those who call evil good, and good evil; Who substitute darkness for light and light for darkness; Who substitute bitter for sweet and sweet for bitter!" (Isaiah 5:20) Everything God has set as a model has become corrupted, perverted and assaulted. Laws are being created to protect the lies and liars yet those who tell the truth are being persecuted.

We can see this evidence from the first chapter in the Bible as Satan immediately attacked everything God created, ruined the natural order and perverted all things to try to create a one-world system where he will be worshiped. God's basic institutions of marriage, families, church and government are all under diabolical attack.

Sin entered the world with the Fall of Adam (Genesis 3) and it distorted the natural relationship between man and woman. This can be clearly seen in the battle of the sexes. Satan's strategy is clear: destroy the family and the created function of men and women. The fall of man began in the Garden of Eden when Adam and Eve sinned. This brought the sin curse on all of creation. Sin is evident everywhere you look. Just look at the news filled with death, looting, murder and all manner of corruption. Despicable acts are committed every day and are getting more and more fervent in tempo.

Just look at a child. Everybody thinks children are innocent, but as soon as they start to move purposefully and utter their first few words they begin to rebel and need correction. You do not have to teach them to resist, to disobey or to lie—you constantly must tell them "No!" and "Stop!" Their first inclinations are fighting, breaking, hurting and lying. Who taught them how to do that? No one, because it was inherent in them due to Adam's sin being passed on through us all. They inherited that through the curse, so we have to teach them to do right in a society that has abandoned morals and principles.

Verses 19-20 tell us *"...because that which is known about God is evident within them; for God made it evident to them. For since the creation of the world His invisible attributes, that is, His eternal power and divine nature, have been clearly perceived, being understood by what has been made, so that they are without excuse."* We can rest assured that we will be without excuse when we stand before our Creator on the last day. God has written His laws on our hearts (the Ten Commandments) and we know what is right and wrong as we were given a conscience—*con* = with; *science* = knowledge or "with knowledge".

Each time we violate our conscience, we violate the God-given truth that is evident within us. It is placed there as a protection. It has been said of some notorious people that have committed horrendous acts "didn't that person have a conscience?" Yes, they did at one time, but each time you violate your conscience, you burn it, making it desensitized so it will not respond so it becomes progressively worse until the conscience is completely burned away and then absolutely despicable acts are committed. Take the sin of sexual lust—it doesn't start out as adultery, rape or murder. It starts out small like lusting after someone, then viewing pornography or using another person for sexual gratification. If left unchecked, it progresses and those things no longer satisfy so it moves to adultery, exposing oneself or becoming a peeping tom, then to rape and so on.

Typically, these progressions of sin are accompanied with guilt so they are drowned with risky behavior such as drinking, drugs and too often, suicide. Sin will always progress in this world but if you are a believer, you must mortify (kill) the flesh; if you are not a believer, please re-read the previous chapter and be reconciled with God today.

Unfortunately, in America many people assume they are "Christians" but they will find themselves in the situation outlined in Matthew 7—God telling them that He never knew them and that they are not welcome. We Americans tend to believe we are on the side of God yet we continue with a lifestyle that is contrary to scripture. We as a nation, and generally in western civilization, have completely abandoned God and no longer have His common grace. *Time* magazine asked if God is dead in April 1966. Since that era, we have removed instruction about the true God from schools and institutions and replaced Him, and thereby morality and truth, for the god of naturalism, paganism and humanism, where everyone is his own authority and his own god.

Verses 21-23 outline this for us in great detail. *"For even though they knew God, they did not honor Him as God or give thanks, but they became futile in their reasonings, and their senseless hearts were darkened. Claiming to be wise, they became fools, and they exchanged the glory of the incorruptible God for an image in the form of corruptible mankind, of birds, four-footed animals, and crawling creatures."* As you can see from this passage, we have removed the true God and have suppressed the truth in unrighteousness, thereby removing ourselves from His blessing and a life that honors Him by helping others.

Verses 24-25 explain that when we abandon God there comes a time when judgment must be fulfilled but common grace still exists: "the rain falls on the just and the unjust" (Matt. 5:45). God has left people who reject Him to their own lusts and evil desires that lead to terrible consequences. In America today, societal restraints have been removed; government and laws cease to function as a protection and sin is allowed to follow after itself leading to destruction. We can see this clearly in our western civilization as lawlessness has overtaken our streets and criminals are not only protected but are eulogized as national heroes, murdering unborn babies is a protected "right", and you are a bigot for not promoting the sexualization of children in the light of LGBTQIA+ agenda.

Back to our Romans passage, we see the progression of decline continues with a sexual revolution, then a homosexual revolution in verses 26-27 and with this sexual homosexual revolution for men it brings a dual punishment on this side of eternity with what could be described as the disease of AIDS and other virulent STIs. Women are mentioned here to reflect the absolute debauchery happening as women are usually the last group to be influenced and to flip from their natural roles but even they fall prey to the dominoes of decline and immorality.

The next section has to be one of the most heartbreaking ones yet, *"And just as they did not see fit to acknowledge God, God gave them up to a depraved mind, to do those things that are not proper,"* scripture says, *"God gave them up to a depraved mind."* A better translation would be "to a reprobate mind," or a mind that cannot function. They have been completely given over in this life—there is no hope for them—they will become victims of their own sin for eternity. We see a similar tale in Exodus with Pharaoh when God sent his messenger Moses to instruct Pharaoh to let the people of God free. Scripture says Pharaoh hardened his heart and God, showing mercy, chastised the people of Egypt for this disobedience with repeated plagues to discipline Pharaoh into compliance. As each plague came about, Pharaoh hardened his heart and would not let the people go. Scripture then says that *God* hardened Pharaoh's heart and at that point it was over for Pharaoh—he had been given over to his sinful desires and it brought him to personal destruction and brought upon Egypt a curse that exists to this day. Do not be like Pharaoh—humble yourself before God, diligently seek Him and you will find Him (Isaiah 55:6).

Verse 29 begins with *"being filled with all unrighteousness, wickedness, greed, evil, full of envy, murder, strife, deceit, malice. They are gossips, slanderers, haters of God and slant, arrogant, boastful, inventors of evil, disobedient to parents, without understanding, untrustworthy, unloving and unmerciful."* All you need to do is spend five minutes watching the news or looking at anything on social media and you can see the absolute filth that is running over in our society. There is absolutely no respect for authority or human life. Light is dark and dark is light.

We now come to the final piece in verse 32: *"And although they knew the ordinance of God that those who practice such things are worthy of death, they not only do the same, but give hardy approval to those who practice them."* As we have seen in verse 28, these reprobates have been given over to a depraved mind. Not only that but in verse 32, they advocate for all these wicked things because they do the same. We can see this all over the news, especially in the last few years.

Look at the depravity of the feminist movement that went from giving women "equal rights" and "voting rights" to now giving on-demand abortion, no questions-asked sexual accusations that ruin the lives of others and an abdication of normal roles as wives and mothers. It is no longer uncommon to see women (and men!) marching around with graphically perverted pink hats, some wearing displays of sexual organs and even acting out the murder of unborn children in bloody detail. It was not very long ago that these sorts of displays would put people in jail or a mental institution but now they are celebrated. Now there are laws passed to protect the devilishly insane and, in fact, to legalize this insanity.

SPIRITUAL CONCLUSIONS

There is no one good; there is no one that seeks after God. If you are not in Christ, even your best intentions are wicked because they are for your own benefit and not the will of God. Simply, we either do the will of God or do the will of Satan.

Now that we have this understanding and solid foundation, I pray that you are saved so you can see through a clear and correct filter. Truth is in Scripture and not in the world. Only through the Bible and Holy Spirit can you can see the motivation of the world system and why things are so bad. Evil men will just continue to become more evil (2 Tim. 3:13). If you are a Christian, you are *in* the world, but not *of* the world. We are not to be preoccupied by earthly things and we will not be ignorant of Satan and his devices. Utilize your critical thinking and do not fall prey to these satanic deceptions.

We have blindly given our autonomy, our children, our health and our freedom over to others in the world system. Sadly, with limited exceptions, our food system is the same. Our food is almost totally out of our control now because we gave it up for convenience to pursue other interests. Almost everything in the market is produced by a handful of companies which are owned by chemical companies, which in turn are owned by pharmaceutical companies, which in turn are owned by the media and banks. It is all one giant corporation with government protection to keep us sick, obese, ignorant and dependent on them, without question.

But it is time to break that cycle—you must utilize critical thinking. Be discerning in everything. Take back your autonomy. Take charge of your health. Take charge of your education and that of your children. Raise your family with multigenerational discipline, wisdom and righteousness.

Before you continue to the next chapter, examine yourself. Do you serve God or do you serve Satan? After answering this question for yourself, you must ask it of these other companies and organizations, especially the government. Examine their motives and their intentions, knowing it is not for your well-being but for their personal gain. If you have been paying attention for any length of time you can start to see that we have been lied to countless times by every entity, including the government, sometimes in complicity *with* the government!

A FINAL THOUGHT ON THE EDUCATION SYSTEM

This is a little off topic, but I would like to address the crisis in our schools. I would like to commend parents that are standing up for their rights at PTA meetings, school board meetings and so on. But, while I applaud their effort, I believe they need to turn that reflection in on themselves. The school board leaders are just going along with the world's satanic system. It is not the responsibility of the state or the government to educate, discipline or provide a moral compass to your children. That responsibility is the *sole* responsibility of the parent; we have relinquished that control to the government and now they have established state indoctrination camps (public schools) and provided protection for themselves at the detriment of our children and our societal future.

It is your responsibility to raise God-fearing, well-educated children through multigenerational wisdom, discipline and knowledge. Again, I commend you for standing up, but it is going to take a lot more than talk. You are going to have to forego some pleasures in the form of vacations, toys, a giant house, new cars, etc. None of these things matter in the long run and your children are the most important job and legacy you have. The schools get paid by how many rumps are in seats. Take that power back, hit them where it hurts...in the wallet.

The next time you are at one of these meetings, instead of venting at the satanic leaders of schools, turn around to your fellow parents, rally together and get your kids out of there!!! The system is irreparably broken, stop sending your kids off to the Devil's playground and expecting angels to come home.

PART TWO:

SAVE YOUR BODY & MIND

- 2 -

KNOW YOUR ENEMY

Pharmaceutical companies and food corporations profit billions of dollars yet when they are caught selling harmful products that have hurt or even killed people, they pay out a pittance settlement to their victims—or their heirs—and then continue practicing the same things under new labels or protections. If you and I were to do something like this, it would be a federal offense. But since these entities are all part of the same system—the right and left hand of the same organism—they protect each other. The collateral damage and injury they cause the consumer is just a part of doing business.

In this section, we will look at some of the devices these corporations employ and the tools they use to oppress us. Do not take my word for it but use these resources, do your own research and take charge of your own health. Do not place your life, or more importantly, your soul, in the hands of a corporate system that wants to destroy you.

MASS-PRODUCED FOOD

The supermarket is a toxic wasteland. At your local chain store, almost everything is full of toxic chemicals such as carcinogens, pesticides, insecticides, herbicides, rodenticides and fungicides— even petroleum products and plastics! And now the powers-that-be want to put mRNA vaccines in some of our most basic and nutrition-dense foods. They have already figured out how to get mRNA vaccines into meat and dairy and now the University of California – Riverside has engineered a lettuce plant with the mRNA vaccine built in. Most of us do not cook lettuce so this raw vegetable will contain an intact mRNA vaccine…

This inability to destroy something genetically implanted in our food is very likely the motive behind vaccine-pusher Bill Gates and his new "Apeel" vegetable coating. This novel synthetic vegetable coating is almost certainly for the sole preservation of the vaccine because all the foods that have this special coating are foods that you would not cook prior to consumption.

Things have gotten so bad that even if you find some decent organic and non-GMO vegetables, all of our fields have been so depleted they are absolutely bereft of any nutritional value. The same field has almost certainly been planted with the same crop for decades. If farmers followed the biblical model of crop rotation and let the land rest, the land would nourish itself and nutrients would be brought back in. As it is now, all the produce is almost completely void of any significant nutrients—with few essential vitamins and few essential minerals. On top of that, they are contaminated inside and out with toxic chemicals from fertilizer, pesticides and more.

We can see the massive issues this has caused by the steady decline in nutrition and the complimentary parallel of malnutrition and chronic disease plaguing the American population. The downgrade in our health parallels the decline of the family after World War II as well. The twentieth century feminist movement was concocted by corporate leaders to get women out of the house to join the workforce, after seeing the model of women working men's jobs during the war. With women both out of the house and in the workforce, "convenience foods" started to roll out. At first, like everything, convenience foods seemed like a good idea but they too were perverted by greed and control.

In the 1970's, during the gas crisis, there was a major push to make ethanol. But as the gas prices dropped, a huge glut of corn sugar was left. That is when the corporations began to petition for the use of high fructose corn syrup. With this booming cash crop, there was a need to protect corn sales, which led to the mass use of industrial herbicides. To bring more profits, they started tampering with God's creation and started genetically modifying many plants with corn being the most common.

A REAL CORNUNDRUM

Currently, the most prevalent, dangerous and genetically modified toxic offender is corn. Corn is used in multitudinous products, including use as thickening and sweetening agents, as well as products such as toothpaste, makeup and even diapers. See list below.

134 CORN SOURCES AND ALTERNATE NAMES

1. Acetic Acid
2. Alcohol
3. Alpha Tocopheral
4. Artificial Flavoring
5. Artificial Sweetener
6. Ascorbate
7. Ascorbic Acid (Vitamin C)*
8. Aspartame
9. Baking Powder
10. Blended Sugar
11. Cake
12. Calcium Citrate
13. Calcium Fumarate
14. Calcium Gluconate
15. Calcium Lactate
16. Calcium Stearate
17. Caramel
18. Caramel Coloring
19. Candy
20. Canned Fruit
21. Cellulose Microcrystalline
22. Cereal
23. Citrus Cloud Emulsion
24. Confectioner's Sugar
25. Cookies
26. Corn
27. Corn Alcohol
28. Corn Gluten
29. Corn Extract
30. Cornflour
31. Cornmeal
32. Cornstarch
33. Corn Oil
34. Corn Oil Margarine
35. Corn Sweetener
36. Corn Sugar
37. Corn Syrup
38. Crystalline Dextrose
39. Dextrin
40. Dextrose
41. D-Gluconic Acid
42. Distilled White Vinegar
43. Erythritol
44. Ethanol
45. Ferrous Gluconate
46. Flavorings
47. Food Starch
48. Fructose
49. Fruit Juice Concentrate
50. Gluconate
51. Glucose
52. Glucose syrup
53. Glutamate
54. Gluten
55. Glycerides
56. Golden Syrup
57. Gravy
58. Grits
59. High-Fructose Corn Syrup (HFCS, HFCS 42, HFCS 55)
60. Hominy
61. Hydrolyzed Corn
62. Hydrolyzed Corn Protein
63. Hydrolyzed Vegetable Protein
64. Ice Cream
65. Infant Formula
66. Inositol
67. Invert Sugar
68. Invert Syrup
69. Iodized Salt
70. Jam
71. Jelly
72. Ketchup
73. Lactate
74. Lactic Acid
75. Lauryl Glucoside
76. Lecithin
77. Linoleic Acid
78. Lysine
79. Maize
80. Malt
81. Malt Extract
82. Malt Syrup
83. Maltitol
84. Maltodextrin
85. Maltose
86. Mannitol
87. Masa Harina
88. Mayonnaise
89. Methyl Glucose
90. Modified Cellulose Gum
91. Modified Corn Starch
92. Modified Food Starch
93. Molasses
94. Monosodium Glutamate
95. MSG
96. Natural Flavorings
97. Olestra/Olean
98. Polenta
99. Polydextrose
100. Polysorbates (i.e. Polysorbate 80)
101. Popcorn
102. Potassium Citrate
103. Potassium Gluconate
104. Powdered Cellulose
105. Powdered Sugar
106. Processed Food
107. Pudding
108. Saccharin
109. Salad Dressing
110. Semolina
111. Soda
112. Sodium Citrate
113. Sodium Erythorbate
114. Sodium Starch Glycolate
115. Sorbate
116. Sorbic Acid
117. Sorbitan
118. Sorbitol
119. Splenda
120. Starch
121. Stearic Acid
122. Sucralose
123. Sucrose
124. Sugar
125. Sweet 'N Low
126. Syrup
127. Unmodified Starch
128. Vegetable Gum Protein
129. Vegetable Paste
130. Vegetable Starch
131. Xanthan Gum
132. Xylitol
133. Yeast
134. Zea Mays

AGUTSYGIRL.COM

What is the big problem with corn? It has been corrupted with *Bacillus thuringiensis*, or Bt. Even a cursory review of just the Wikipedia page on Bt says the mode of action is gut paralysis, although they are quick to note, without support, that it does not affect humans.

Bt is basically forcing a fungus gene into the corn genome so that when insects eat the corn it paralyzes their guts and makes pores in their intestines. (Remember, "pore" = hole.) This is what is causing our epidemic of "leaky gut." From the charts, it is easy to see the skyrocketing increase in allergies and other ailments after the introduction of GMO corn. Autism rates are exponential, chronic illnesses are off the charts, and allergies have taken over the masses. GMO's and Bt will be further discussed in a future chapter.

THE RISE IN MYSTERIOUS CHRONIC ILLNESS

In the next few chapters, we will explore "mysterious" chronic illness and the allergies epidemic that has come about since the early 1990's. Most of these illnesses were present before but now have been wildly exacerbated by genetic tampering, excessive toxins, vaccines and other manipulative agents.

These issues all come back to the pyramid scheme of American government working hand in glove with a few mega-corporations (all tied back to banking and pharmaceuticals) and being under the total control of a handful of globalist elites bent on world domination. The Bible says that "the love of money is the root of all evil" and that has never been more evident in western civilization than it is now. The media, government and big business lie and tell us their products and services are safe so they can make money. When their dangerous practices become too obvious to hide, they pay out a paltry settlement to the survivors and by then they have replaced that deadly product for another.

Take the health care system in the United States—we have the most expensive healthcare in the world and yet we also have the highest amount of chronic illness and the lowest longevity in an industrialized nation. Following are some statistics from the hospital industry:

- Medical billing errors cost Americans $210,000,000,000 annually.
- Roughly 12,000,000 Americans are misdiagnosed each year.
- Medical errors cause an estimated 250,000-440,000 deaths in the United States annually.
- As many as 80% of medical bills contain at least one error.
- A little more than 4,000 surgical errors occur each year.
- It is estimated that 7,000 to 9,000 patients die every year from medication errors.
- Medical error is the 3rd leading cause of death in America.

(Source: *mymedicalscore.com*)

Top Ten Causes of Death in the United States (2016)

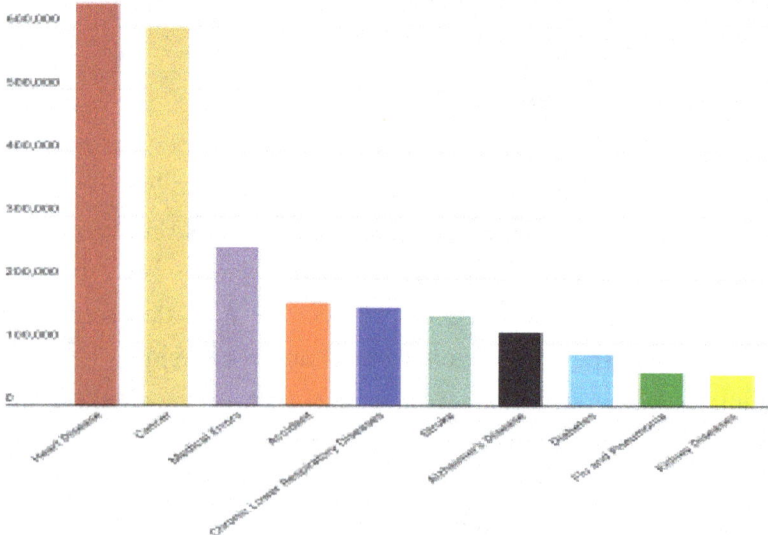

These are the "experts" you are blindly trusting with your life.

If you or your loved one are diagnosed with any health issue, you must do your own research or you risk being one of the twelve million Americans that are misdiagnosed. There could be a natural health remedy for your condition instead of petroleum-based medications that only mask symptoms while causing more conditions, that in turn need more "treatment."

Doctors are not trained to treat the cause of your condition—or even basic nutrition—they are taught to be nothing more than a white-collar drug dealer for which they get massive kickbacks. The *Physician's Desk Reference* (*PDR* – now a digital app) is a large book every doctor has. The *PDR* contains over 250,000 medications and, apart from a few antibiotics, none of the medications actually *cure* any disease. Doctors, hospitals and pharmaceutical companies do not make more money if you are cured so there has not been a cure for a disease for over sixty years.

Like everything in our world today, your body and life are now on a subscription plan. All the facets of food, drugs, lifestyle and control are to make us weak, sick, ignorant and dependent on the elites for everything. During the Covid-19 "pandemic," hospitals were incentivized to do testing and to alter long-standing protocols and procedures. They quickly and radically changed protocols and started intubating people as a first-line defense when in reality, a ventilator is normally a last-ditch effort to save someone's life. But hospitals were being paid an additional $13,000 – $39,000 per patient for positive Covid-19 cases and ventilator use. In some cases, they were being paid up to $55,000 for each Covid-19 submission and extra pay when Covid-19 was listed as the cause of death. This means car crash victims or other non-illness related deaths were still a payout for hospitals if the victim simply tested positive for Covid-19.

Covid-19 testing itself has come under great scrutiny as the tests are giving false positives at a rate far outside an acceptable margin of error. As you may well know, the "pandemic" was not about a viral infection that had a 99.889% survivability rate, it was all about control and isolating power among the few. If we had already had a digital, cashless society in place, we would have never been able to recover from becoming a totalitarian régime during the plandemic. The powers-that-be are working to solve that problem with the FedNow banking system in which your every transaction is now handled and tracked by the government—another topic for your own research.

Another part of the overall American puzzle is the Illusion of Choice. Everything from the supermarket to the evening news to social media is controlled by a handful of companies that have government protection and get their orders straight from the government. The CIA admitted decades ago to "Operation Mockingbird" in which they have placed agents in *every* media outlet in America. After the repeal of the Smith-Mundt Act in 2012, it is now legal for the government to propagandize its own citizens and give protection for the media outlets that parrot their lies. There are considerable video montages of media personalities from all over the country, robotically chanting exact scripted lines: "…this is extremely dangerous for our democracy…" Why would this happen in a free and constitutionally protected nation unless there was an agenda behind it?

The government and their media lackeys also condition our responses by selectively leaking bits of stories over long periods of time so that when the truth comes out it is not a shock—it sounds familiar and is overlooked as old news. Following are several charts that show the Illusion of Choice and how our entire system is controlled by a select few.

Shut Up & Die

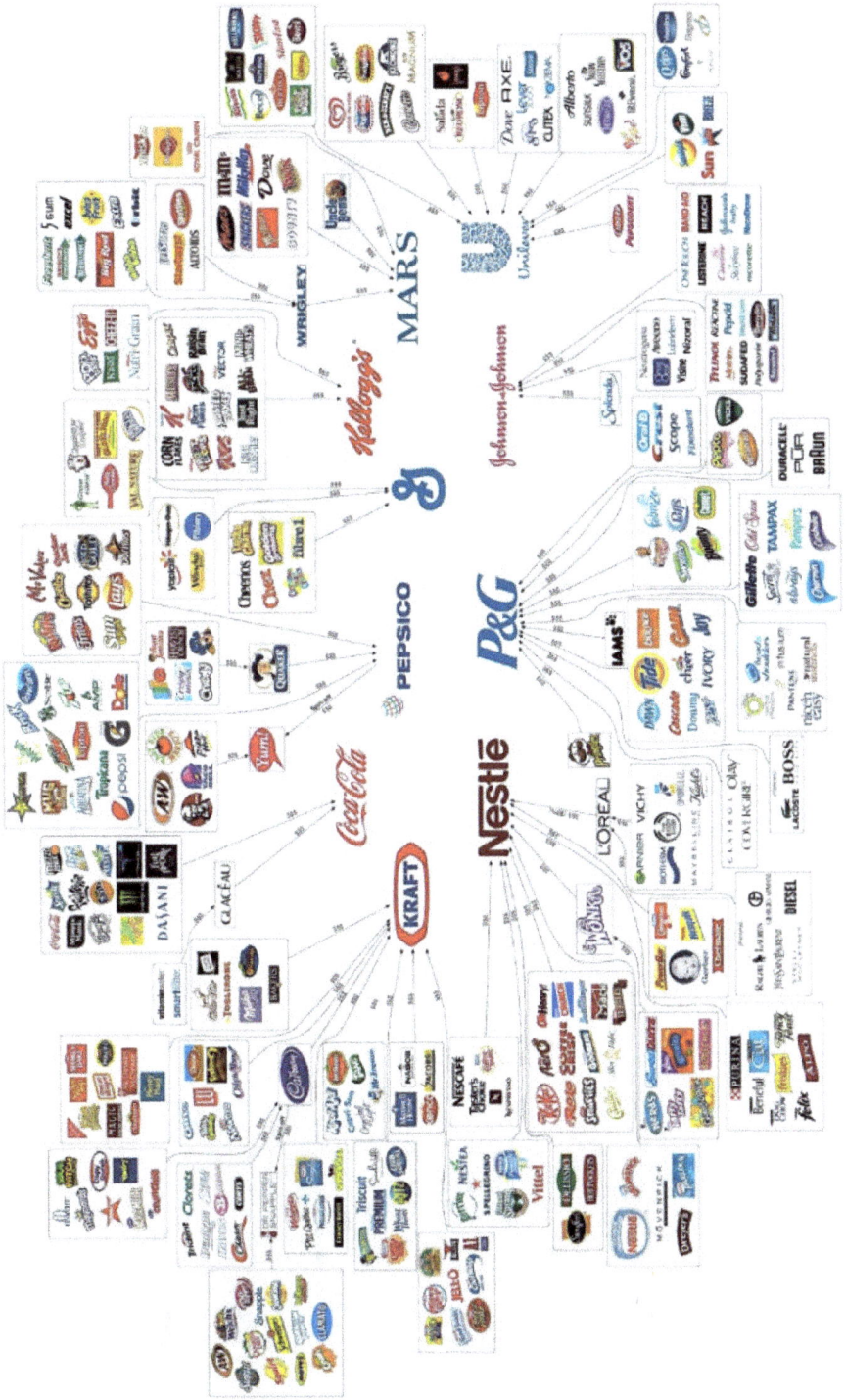

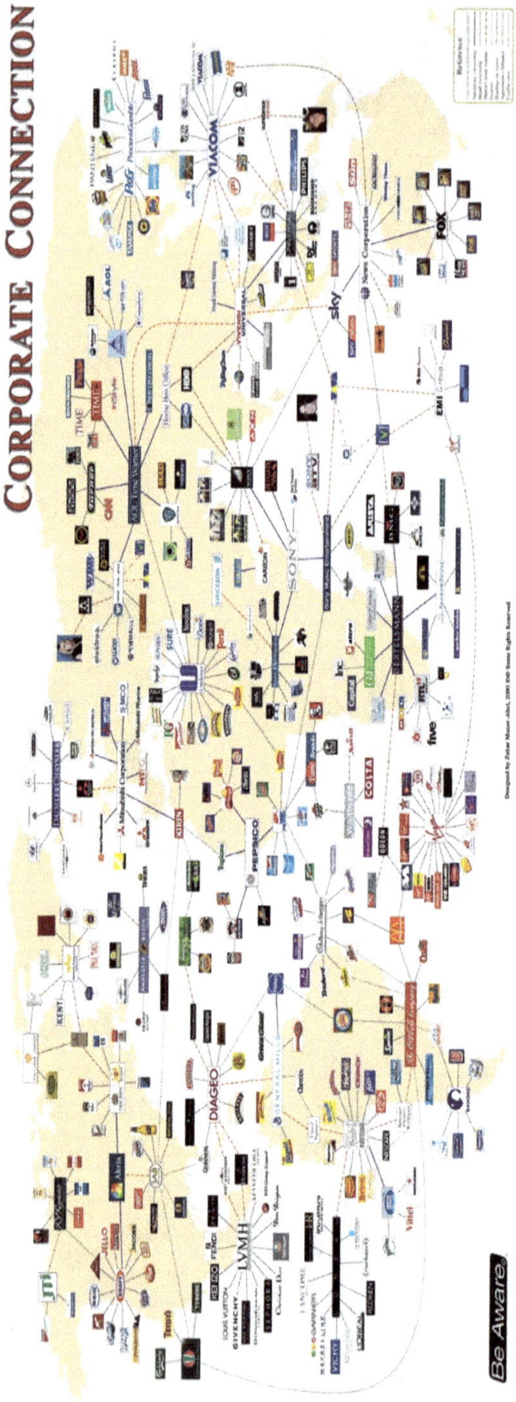
CORPORATE CONNECTION
VIACOM
AOL Time Warner
SONY
BERTELSMANN
News Corporation
FOX
PEPSICO
DIAGEO
LVMH
Be Aware

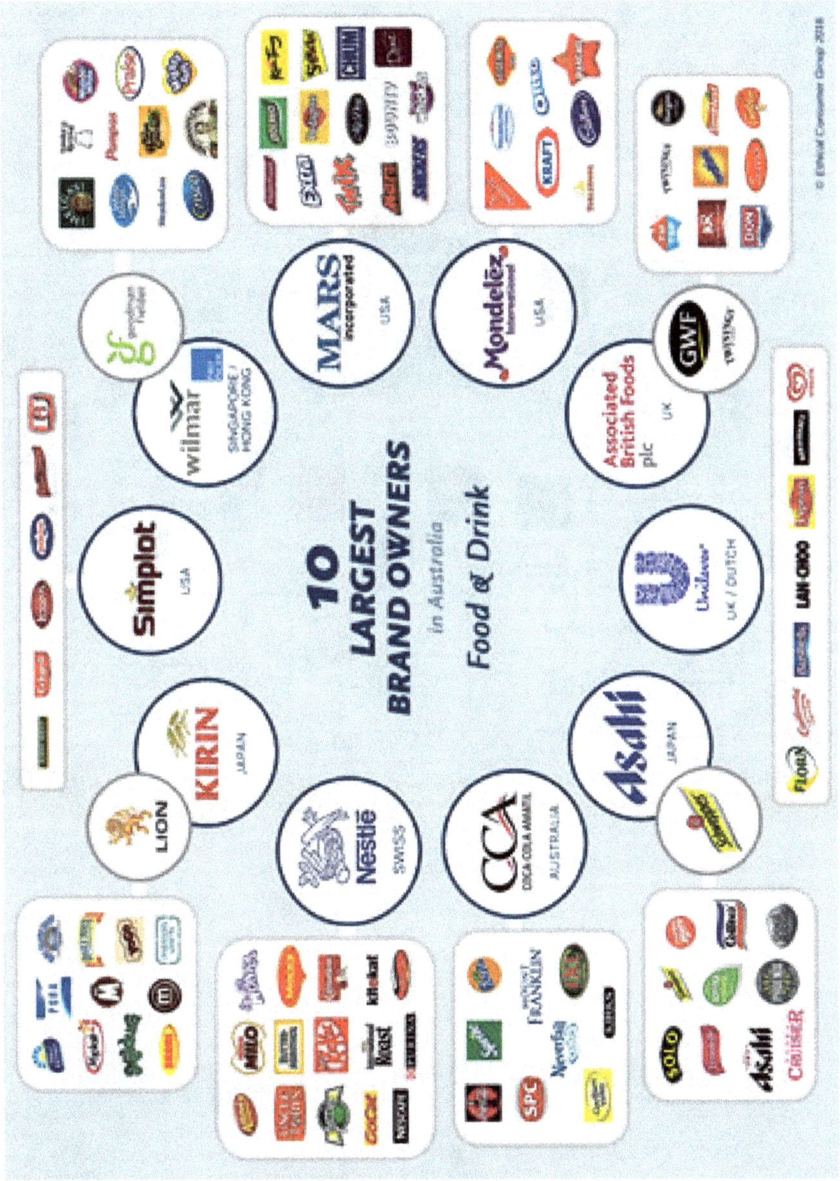
10
LARGEST
BRAND OWNERS
in Australia
Food & Drink
Simplot
USA
KIRIN
JAPAN
LION
wilmar
SINGAPORE / HONG KONG
MARS
incorporated
USA
Mondelēz
USA
Associated British Foods plc
UK
GWF
Unilever
UK / DUTCH
Asahi
JAPAN
CCA
AUSTRALIA
Nestlé
SWISS

THE WEB WORLD
WHO
OWNS WHO?

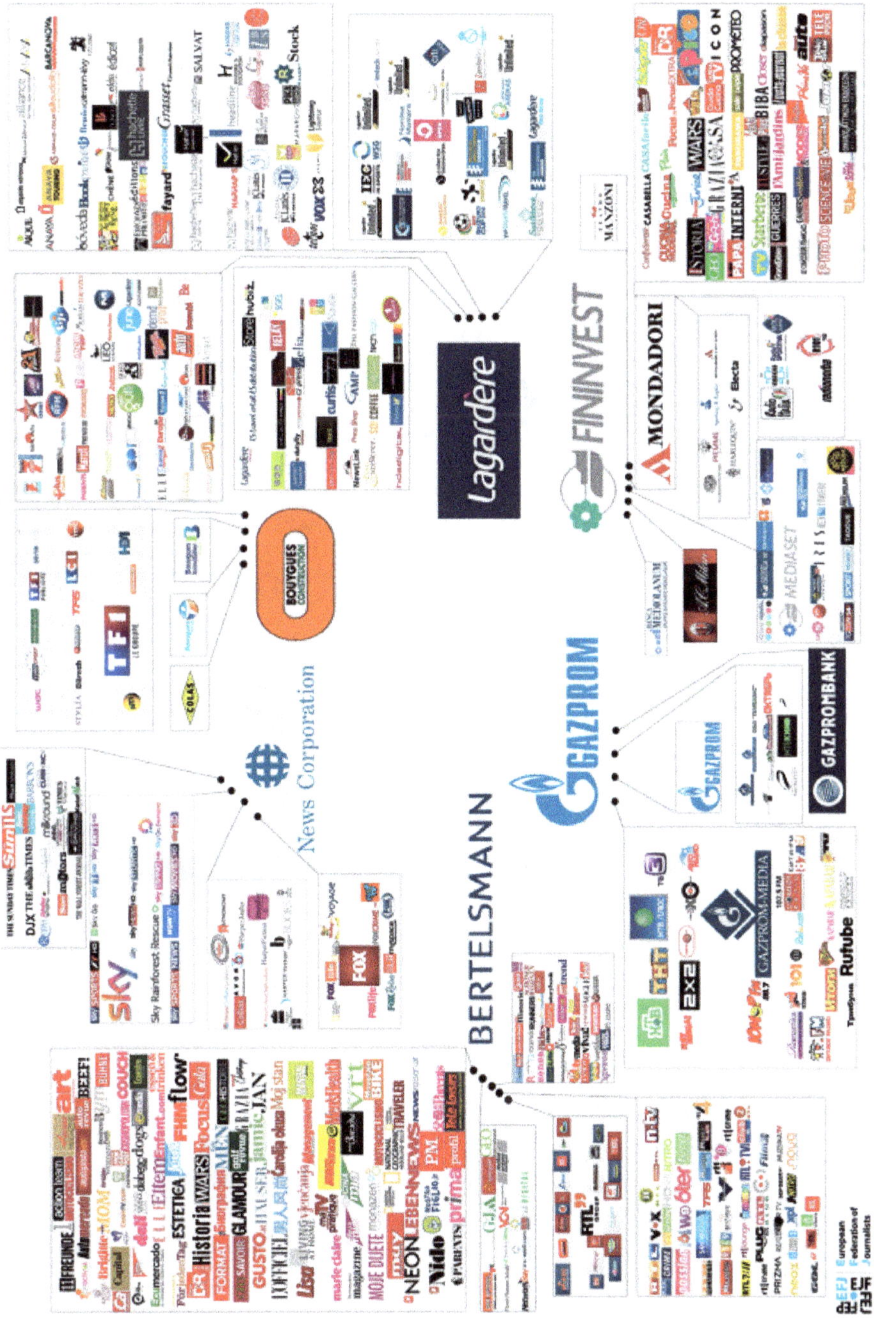

Lagardère
FININVEST
MONDADORI
MEDIASET
GAZPROM
GAZPROMBANK
GAZPROM-MEDIA
Rutube
BERTELSMANN
News Corporation
FOX
sky
BOUYGUES CONSTRUCTION
TF1
COLAS
MANZONI
EFJ European Federation of Journalists

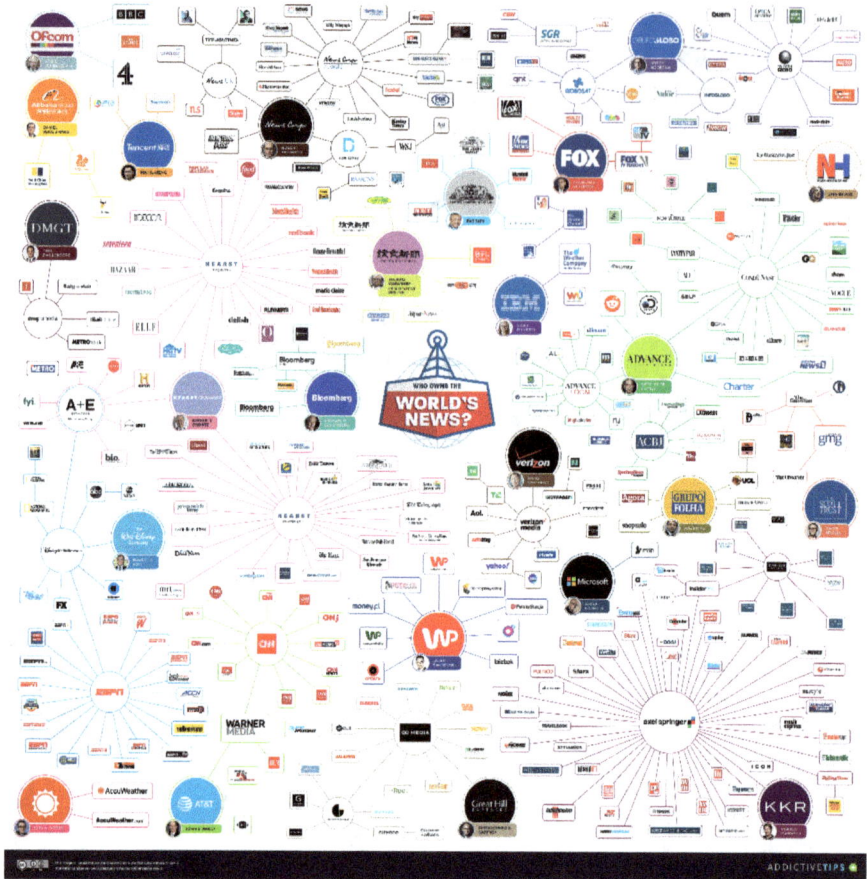

Chart Sources:

www.infographicnow.com/lifestyle/food/food-infographic-infograph-shows-how-just-10-companies-own-all-the-worlds-food-brands/

www.lifecoachcode.com/2017/02/02/companies-own-food-media-internet/

www.ethical.org.au/consumer/map7/chart7.htm

www.visualcapitalist.com/internet-giants-owns-web/

FOLLOW THE MONEY – THE ROTHSCHILDS

We can see the evidence of the global control that banks have over nations by examining the largest banking dynasty in history – the Rothschilds. This dynasty got its start in 1743 when a goldsmith named Amschel Moses Bauer opened a coin shop in Frankfurt, Germany. The sign that hung outside his shop was a red shield depicting a Roman eagle. His shop was known as the Red Shield Firm. Amschel taught his son, Meyer Amschel Bauer, everything about business, from money lending to finance. Meyer worked for the Oppenheimers as a clerk in their bank in Hannover. His brilliance was well-received and his success allowed him to purchase his father's firm after his father died. The red shield still hung outside his father's firm, so he adopted the red shield as his logo and changed his surname to Rothschild. In German, "Rot" means red and "Schild" means shield, giving us "Red Shield".)

Meyer's experience with the Oppenheimers had taught him it was far more lucrative and beneficial to loan money to governments and kings instead of private citizens. Meyer taught his five sons (Amschel, Salomon, Nathan, Karl and Jacob) the family business of creating money and manipulating governments. He sent his sons to open branches in the major capital cities of Europe: Amschel to Frankfurt, Nathan to London, Karl to Naples, and Jacob to Paris.

Today, the Rothschilds still hold the purse strings to most major governments and have been instrumental in the establishment of many nefarious persons, policies and institutions. This kind of backroom, members-only manipulation still continues today as most of our government officials are related to or have ties back to these events and families through one channel or another.

The Rothschilds have had their fingers on the pulse of world events for centuries. They were heavily involved with a man named Adam Weishaupt, who founded the Illuminati in 1776, which later infiltrated the newly founded United States. They were also part of the secret meeting at Jekyll Island in 1910 where the Federal Reserve was concocted. Please note that the so-called Federal Reserve is NOT actually part of the United States federal government. Also at this meeting was Paul Warburg. Paul's wife was from the Kuhn, Loeb & Co. banking family and his brother-in-law was Jacob Schiff, whose father (Moses Schiff) worked for the Rothschilds. Jacob went on to loan empires the money they needed for war efforts in the twentieth century. Jacob Schiff's heritage almost certainly includes US Representative Adam Schiff and another descendent was married to Al Gore's daughter. With just cursory research, it is clear that our "leaders" are an incestuous cesspool.

Here are a few choice quotes from Nathan Rothschild:

"Permit me to issue and control the money of a nation, and I care not who makes the laws."

"I care not what puppet is placed upon the throne of England to rule the Empire on which the sun never sets. The man who controls the British money supply controls the British Empire, and I control the British money supply."

With elusive puppet-masters pulling the strings from behind the scenes, the illusion of choice becomes all the murkier and harder to discern but we must push through to see the truth and act accordingly.

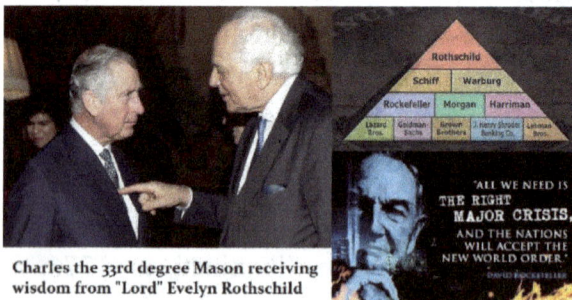

Charles the 33rd degree Mason receiving wisdom from "Lord" Evelyn Rothschild

- 3 -

TRADITIONAL vs MODERN FARMING PRACTICES

Proper farming practices should generally model the biblical mandate given in Exodus 23:10-11. The reason for crop rotation is so that the land will not become void of vital nutrients later in the food cycle—for animal and human consumers. When rotation is properly implemented, the parcels of land cycle crops, and even animals, to infuse (and sometimes to remove) different nutrients back into the matrix to benefit both the plant's hardiness and harvest potential as well as the plant-consumers, whether they be for meat animals or directly for human consumption.

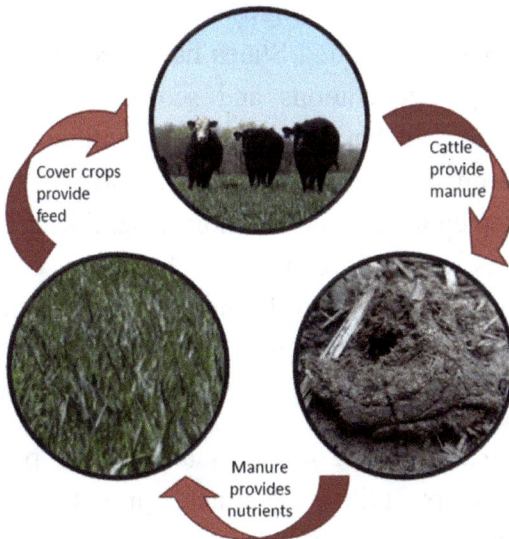

(Photo Source cropwatch.unl.edu)

Basic Crop Rotation

Lettuce, arugula, kale, swiss chard, spinach, cabbage, etc.

Green beans, edamame, dried beans, cowpeas, lentils, etc.

Leaf

Legume

Root

Fruit

Carrots, onions, beets, radish, potatoes, parsnips, sweet potatoes, etc.

The Seasonal Homestead

Tomatoes, summer squash, winter squash, cucumbers, peppers, etc.

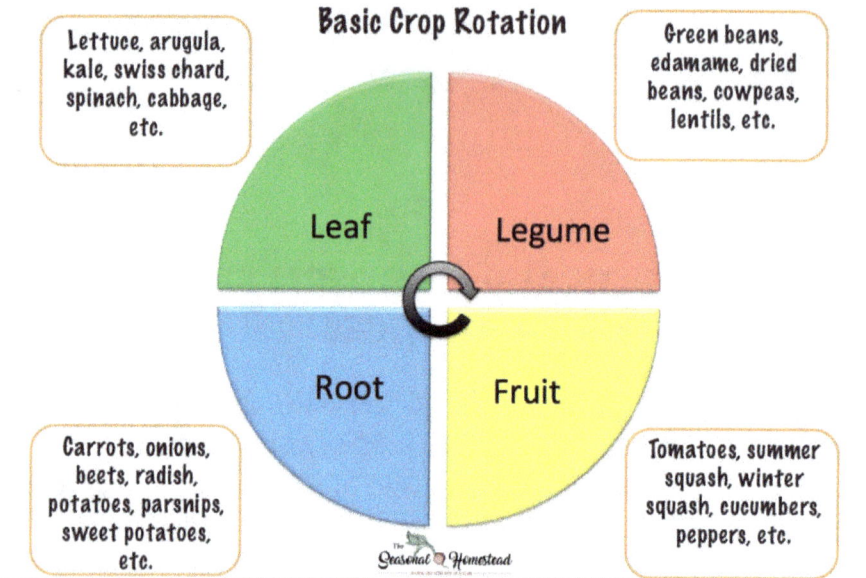

(Source: theseasonalhomestead.com)

HOW NUTRITIOUS IS YOUR PRODUCE?

The modern farming method does use an over-simplified model of crop rotation but without the highly important natural revitalization process. Farms in the United States have been growing the same crop for multiple generations and scores, maybe hundreds, of years—a few farms in America have been continuously in operation for over three hundred years. The vast majority of our farms have completely depleted the land of most essential minerals and the produce that is grown is completely bereft of vital minerals in beneficial amounts. Very few farms ever replace the minerals in their fields—the only supplementation is petroleum-based fertilizer that makes the plants grow, regardless of their nutritional content.

In addition to the lack of nutrients and use of petroleum-based fertilizers, farmers utilize chemical insecticides, pesticides, fungicides, herbicides, rodenticides and plant growth factor.

Mineral Depletion in Our Soil

Source: USDA (US Department of Agriculture)

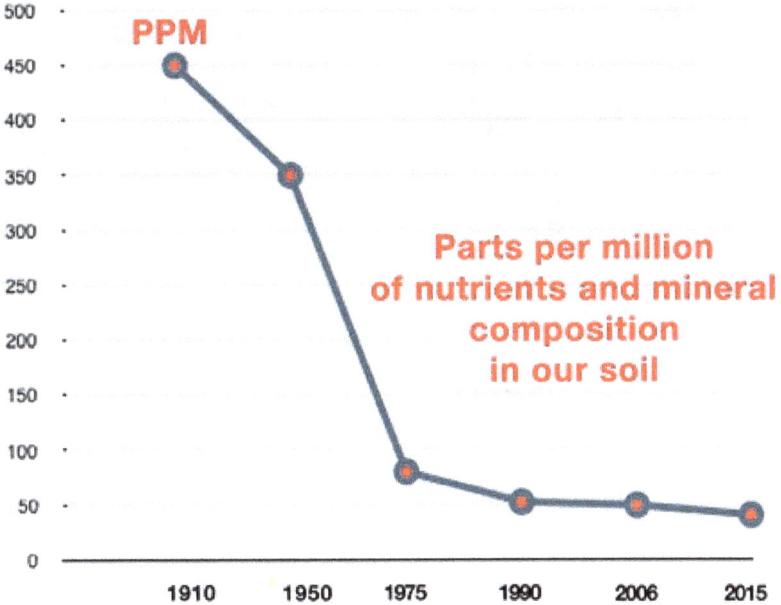

PPM

**Parts per million
of nutrients and mineral
composition
in our soil**

1953

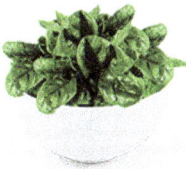

Iron
Content

1997

=

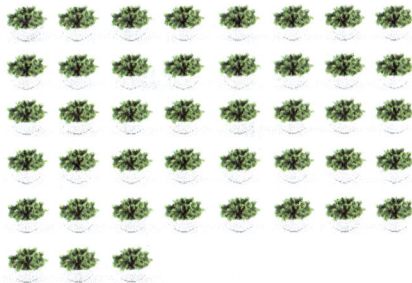

(Source: turtlemountainblog.com/soil-depletion-and-the-ucla-spinach-study-
what-you-need-to-know/0

35

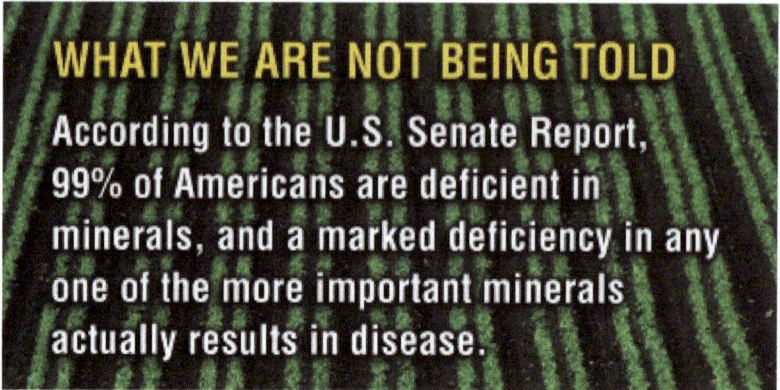

WHAT WE ARE NOT BEING TOLD

According to the U.S. Senate Report, 99% of Americans are deficient in minerals, and a marked deficiency in any one of the more important minerals actually results in disease.

(Source: www.strongbrain365.blogspot.com/2015/06/soil-depletion-and-mental-health.html)

A US national survey, NHANES 2007-2010, which surveyed 16,444 individuals four years and older, reported a high prevalence of inadequacies for multiple micronutrients (see Table 1). Specifically, the US population does not meet the daily requirement for:

- 94.3% for vitamin D
- 88.5% for vitamin E
- 52.2% for magnesium
- 44.1% for calcium
- 43.0% for vitamin A
- 38.9% for vitamin C

For the nutrients in which a daily value requirement has not been set:

- 100% for potassium
- 91.7% for choline
- 66.9% for vitamin K

The prevalence of inadequacies was low for all the B vitamins and several minerals, including copper, iron, phosphorus, selenium, sodium, and zinc (see Table 1). These are just some of the nutrients listed but we actually need ninety essential minerals and vitamins. Some are extremely vital and are depleted by our diet, toxins and heavy metals stored in the body. We will go over basic nutrition and supplementation in another chapter.

Table 1 – Nutritional Inadequacies

Inadequacies Among US Residents Ages ≥4 Years (26)		
Micronutrient	Mean Daily Intake from Food*	% < EAR
Folate	542 µg DFE	9.5
Niacin	24.7 mg	1.1
Riboflavin	2.2 mg	2.1
Thiamin	1.6 mg	4.7
Vitamin A	621 µg RAE	43.0
Vitamin B_6	2.0 mg	9.5
Vitamin B_{12}	5.3 µg	2.5
Vitamin C	84.0 mg	38.9
Vitamin D	4.9 µg	94.3
Vitamin E[#]	7.4 mg	88.5
Vitamin K	85.2 µg	66.9[†]
Calcium	987 mg	44.1
Copper	1.3 µg	4.2
Iron	15.1 mg	7.4
Magnesium	286 mg	52.2
Phosphorus	1,350 mg	1.0
Potassium	2,595 mg	100[†]
Selenium	108 µg	0.3
Sodium	3,433 mg	0.1[†]
Zinc	11.7 mg	11.7
Choline[††]	315 mg	91.7[†]

(Source: www.lpi.oregonstate.edu/mic/micronutrient-inadequacies/overview)

- 4 -

GMO's: THE MISSING LINK

With recent scrutiny of GMO's or, genetically engineered organisms, the food and chemical industries have lobbied to have GMO's relabeled as "bioengineered products" and they are throwing a fortune into preventing products from being labeled with clear information. Why is this? Following are charts with the battle lines drawn between companies who want to have GMO's listed on products or not. Pay attention to the players who are against this regulation and what their motives may be.

(Source: www.ordinaryvegan.net)

(Source: www.cornucopia.org)

By now, you should be seeing some recognizable names and patterns. The history of GMO's started in the 1970's and by 1994, there were commercially available GMO products on shelves in the US. When you research GMO's, they have cute charts and explanations that make it sound like this is just a normal process that has taken place over the long history of agriculture. Far from the truth, these seeds are being altered by splicing genes from animals, bacteria and other organisms that could never cross pollinate or breed in nature. Please see Chart 1 for another look.

Chart 1 – What is a GMO?

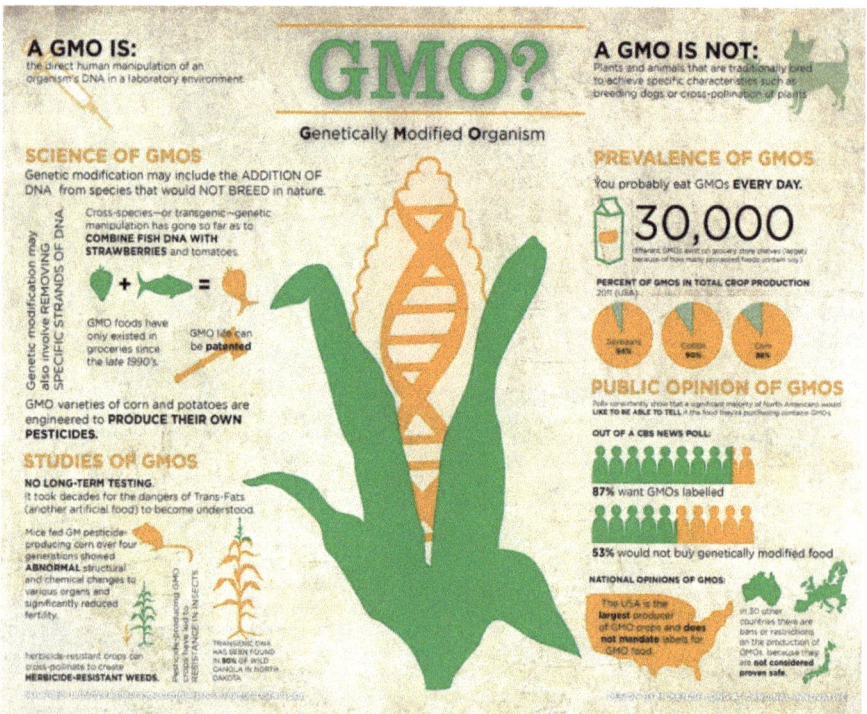

(Source: https://peeltheorange.com/pressroom/gmofactsheet.php)

HOW DO WE GET GMO's?

Crops are modified in 4 different ways to become a genetically modified organism:

1. Mutagenesis – exposing seeds to chemicals or radiation.
2. RNA interference – switching off selected genes with RNA.
3. Transgenetics – inserting genes using recombinant DNA methods.
4. Traditional breeding – cross-pollinating plants—the natural process.

The main culprit of the GMO family is *Bacillus thuringiensis* or Bt. Again, Bt is a soil-dwelling bacterium and the most commonly used biological pesticide worldwide. The mode of action for this biological pesticide—that has been gene-spliced into crops—is that it creates spores that form toxic insecticidal proteins.

The toxic proteins Bt creates insoluble crystals in the guts of a variety of insects and nematodes. The gut breaks this crystal down, which releases the toxin that is then absorbed into the cell membranes of the gut, **"paralyzing the digestive tract and forming a pore."** This action causes the insect to cease eating and quickly starve to death.

(Source: https://en.wikipedia.org/wiki/Bacillus_thuringiensis)

Please pay particular attention to the bolded section: "paralyzing the digestive tract and forming a pore." Using our critical thinking, we can see that whatever organism eats this Bt-modified food will have some paralysis of the digestive tract along with developing holes as well. This sounds exactly like a condition that has come to light since 1994, when GMO's were introduced, called "intestinal permeability" or more commonly, "leaky gut."

Leaky gut has almost certainly been the catalyst for the explosion of chronic illness, allergies, autoimmune disorders and autism. When your digestive tract membranes are porous, your food, waste and any toxins are passed *directly* into the blood stream, causing an autoimmune response. Since GMO's started being mass-produced in 1994, we can look at the explosion of peanut allergies in children from that point forward as a striking example of this issue.

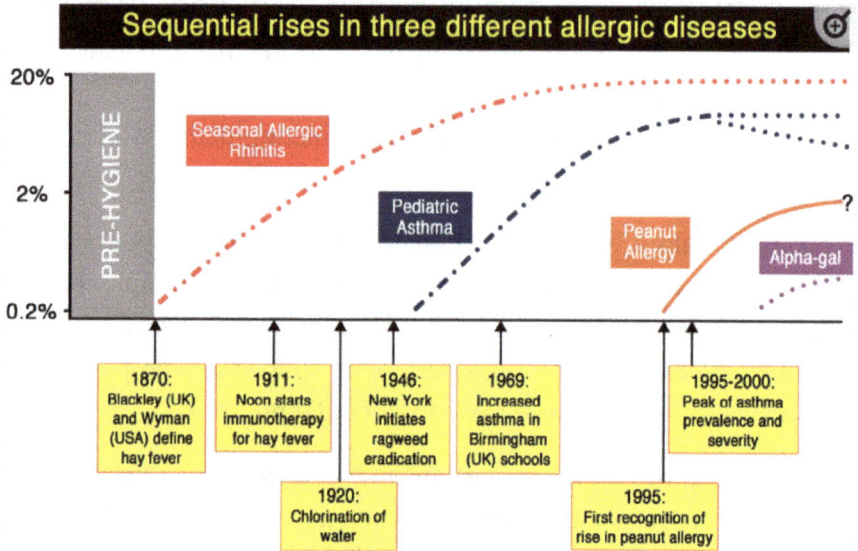

Sequential rises in three different allergic diseases

1870: Blackley (UK) and Wyman (USA) define hay fever	1911: Noon starts immunotherapy for hay fever	1946: New York initiates ragweed eradication	1969: Increased asthma in Birmingham (UK) schools		1995-2000: Peak of asthma prevalence and severity	

1920: Chlorination of water

1995: First recognition of rise in peanut allergy

(Source The Allergy Epidemics: 1870–2010 PMCID: PMC4617537

NIHMSID: NIHMS697397

PMID: 26145982)

THE GMO-ALLERGY CONNECTION

The explanation for the exponential rise in peanut allergies seen in 1995 is the same reason for the explosion of chronic illness and autoimmune disease since that time. Bt causes leaky gut so when you eat foreign proteins, in this case, peanuts, the partially digested peanuts, along with toxins from all the previously-mentioned sources, are passed directly into your blood stream through the holes in the intestines and thereby cause the body to go into attack mode and provoking an immune response to the foreign proteins.

Generations that grew up before the 1990's could hardly remember anyone with food allergies but now school nurse offices are filled with EpiPens at the ready for all the severely allergic kids. Please see the chart above to see that the rise in peanut allergies directly correlates with the introduction of Bt-laden GMO's into our food supply in 1994. This would also explain the explosion in other allergies such as nuts, soy, wheat gluten, dairy, etc. since 1994. Incidentally, the most significant Bt GMO crops include staple produce such as potatoes, corn, sweet corn, eggplant, cotton, rice, tomatoes, sugarcane and soybeans.

GMO-AUTISM CONNECTION

Bt-infused products causing leaky gut, in conjunction with childhood vaccines that contain thimerosal (mercury) as a preservative and commonly containing varying mixtures of aluminum, formalin and cell tissue from aborted babies—have created a chimeric toxic cocktail for your babies and children. Your baby may have developed leaky gut from receiving Bt and GMO filled nutrients directly from its mother in utero.

Research in eastern Quebec in 2011 showed Bt toxins in the blood of pregnant women and that it had indeed passed to the fetus. When the infant is born with leaky gut and is then given multiple doses of vaccines that contain heavy metals (mercury, aluminum, etc.), the body attempts to flush the toxins out through the usual mode of action via the digestive and urinary systems. With a leaky gut, the heavy metals are passed through the pores, into the intestine and directly into the blood stream, causing a severe reaction to the toxic metals and other vaccine ingredients.

Mercury is not only cumulative, but it also crosses the blood-brain barrier to store primarily in the pituitary and hypothalamus—which are vitally important to growth and development. To compound the issue, toxins that are not bonded travel though the bile and the bile is reabsorbed into the liver, creating a toxic cycle (see Chart 2). If you have witnessed a child that became autistic after a round of childhood vaccines, you can clearly see the signs of mercury poisoning. There is a great documentary online called "Vaxxed" for more on the vaccine-connection to autism.

Chart 2 – Bile Circulation Graphic

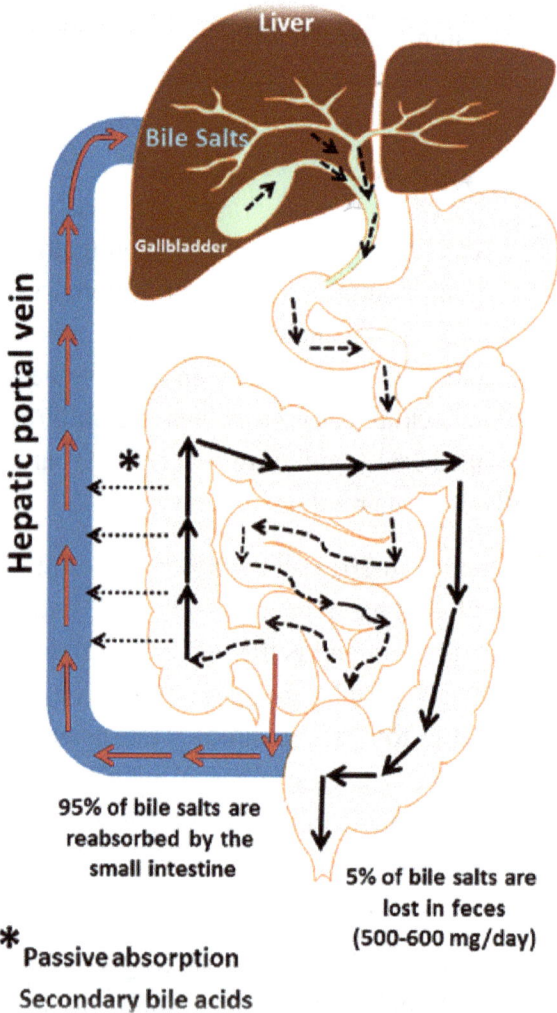

Liver

Bile Salts

Gallbladder

Hepatic portal vein

*

95% of bile salts are reabsorbed by the small intestine

5% of bile salts are lost in feces (500-600 mg/day)

*Passive absorption
Secondary bile acids

https://www.researchgate.net/publication/262193252_Bile_Acids_are_Nutrient_Signaling_Hormones

KNOW THE SIGNS

The following are signs of mercury toxicity:

- Feeling numb or dull pain in certain parts of your body
- Uncontrollable tremors or "Parkinsonism"
- Unsteady walk
- Double vision or blurry vision
- Blindness
- Memory loss
- Seizures
- Burning sensation in your stomach and/or throat
- Nausea or vomiting
- Diarrhea
- Blood in vomit or stool
- Urine color changes
- Coughing
- Trouble breathing
- Metallic taste in your mouth
- Nausea or vomiting
- Bleeding or swollen gums
- Personality Disorders
- Emotional Disturbances
- Mad Hatter Syndrome (Erethism)
- Allergies

Developmental delays in children include:

- Cognition
- Fine motor skills
- Speech and language development
- Visual-spatial awareness
- Hearing and speech difficulties
- Lack of coordination

- Muscle weakness
- Nerve loss in hands and face
- Trouble walking
- Vision changes
- Anxiety
- Depression
- Irritability
- Memory problems
- Numbness of the hands, feet, or mouth
- Pathologic shyness
- Tremors

If you or your loved one, especially a child, is showing these signs, please talk to a functional medicine doctor immediately.

NAVIGATING GMO's

To start to heal you must remove as many GMO foods from your diet as possible—all if you can. This task is getting increasingly more difficult because companies are lobbying to not have to disclose GMO's through labeling and they are successful at getting the names changed to "bioengineering", "biotechnology," etc.

If you want to do further research, here is a list of more organisms that are gene-spliced into our food chain.

- *Escherichia coli* or E. Coli
- *Bacillus thuringiensis* (multiple strains)
- *Corynebacterium glutamicum*
- *Stenotrophomonas maltophilia*
- *Streptomyces viridochromogenes.*

The Official FDA Food GMO timeline says the first product was the 1994 Flavr Savr Tomato by Calgene (later bought out by Monsanto). This is incorrect as they changed FDA guidance protocol in 1992 because of a 1991 letter from Calgene about their Flavr Savr project.

The FDA approved their guidance for domestic/non-domestic cultivation use in 1992. In the Calgene patents, they cite a 1988 study of "Transgenic Tomatoes". Additionally in 1992, the book "Safety Assessment of Genetically Engineered Fruits and Vegetable: A Case Study of the Flavr Savr Tomato" was written by the top researchers at Calgene; just another fox watching over the henhouse situation.

Sources:

www.isaaa.org/gmapprovaldatabase/event/default.asp?EventID=178&Event=FL AVR%SAVR

www.bch.cbd.int/en/database/14867

www.wayback.archive-it.org/7993/20180124124721/https://fda.gov/food/ingredientspackaginglabeling/GEplants/Submissions/ucm225027.htm

GMOs Around the World

18 million farmers grew GMO crops in 2016. Most were from small farms in developing countries.

26 countries grew GMOs in 2016

19 developing countries grew GMOs

7 industrialized countries grew GMOs

As of 2016, GMOs are **GROWN**, **IMPORTED** and/or used in **FIELD TRIALS** in more than **75 countries.**

GROWING BIOTECH AND COUNTING IMPORT APPROVALS
Argentina
Australia
Bangladesh
Bolivia
Brazil
Burkina Faso
Canada
Chile
China
Colombia
Costa Rica
Czech Republic
Honduras
India

Mexico
Myanmar
Pakistan
Paraguay
Philippines
Portugal
Slovakia
South Africa
Spain
Sudan
United States
Uruguay
Vietnam

GRANTING IMPORT APPROVALS
Austria
Belgium
Bolivia
Burkina Faso
Croatia
Cuba
Cyprus
Denmark
Egypt
Estonia
Finland
France
Greece
Hungary
Iran
Israel
Italy
Japan
Latvia

Lithuania
Luxembourg
Malaysia
Malta
Netherlands
New Zealand
Norway
Poland
Russia
Singapore
Slovenia
South Korea
Sweden
Switzerland
Taiwan
Turkey
Wales

APPROVING RESEARCH FIELD TRIALS
Cameroon
Ghana
Ghana
Kenya
Nigeria
Swaziland
Uganda
United Kingdom

In 2016, Spain grew **95%** of all GM corn in the EU

39% of crop area devoted to GMOs globally is in the U.S.

10 countries in Latin America grow GMOs:
Argentina
Bolivia
Brazil
Chile
Colombia
Costa Rica
Honduras
Mexico
Paraguay
Uruguay

Australia first planted GMOs in 1996. In 2015, **94%** of Australia's cotton crop was GMO

India is the **#1** cotton producer in the world. **96%** of India's cotton is GM

3 GM crops are being cultivated in Africa

The public-private partnership **Water Efficient Maize for Africa** is developing drought-tolerant and insect-resistant corn for local farmer use.

- 5 -

PESTICIDE + HERBICIDE + FUNGICIDE + RODENTICIDE = HOMICIDE

Have you or someone you know been diagnosed with a nut, fruit, gluten or dairy intolerance or allergy? It is not the veggies, fruit, nuts, protein and dairy that are making you sick, it is what the producers have done to them. God made them good, and we have destroyed them with our wicked tampering, thereby rendering them devoid of anything nutritional on top of basically poisoning them with chemicals and genetic modifications.

There have been and still are a plethora of toxic chemicals that are applied to our crops that are extremely dangerous. The basics are pesticides (kills bugs), herbicides (kills plants), fungicides (kills fungus, mold), and rodenticides (kills rodents and others).

One of the most insidious of these chemicals was a mercury-based fungicide/pesticide that was used for decades on both crops and as a seed dressing. Most uses have been banned but it still continues to be used as a seed dressing to prevent seed rot. As a result, many fields are loaded with heavy metal residue that leeches into the water supply—we see this in the sugarcane fields in Australia that have leeched into the sea and into the Great Barrier Reef.

The herbicide called *Atrazine* is one of the most used in the United States. It causes such severe endocrine disruptions in frogs that it causes them to morph into females that continuously lay fertile eggs—just image what that is doing to generations of Americans drinking tainted water and having their endocrine systems constantly in flux.

THE MONSANTO PROBLEM

Monsanto is the manufacturer of most GMO seeds and chemicals applied to crops and they own many food brands. We can see from Chart 3 why these companies fight so hard not to have their products labeled as "GMO."

In addition to the GMO's they produce and grow, the crops are sprayed with numerous poisons Monsanto creates as well. You may remember hearing about Agent Orange—they still use one of the main components of Agent Orange called 2,4-D and it is sprayed on our food crops. One of the most prolific Monsanto products is an herbicide called Roundup (composed of glyphosate). It is repeatedly applied to crops and used as an off-label desiccant. The farmers spray crops at the end of the cycle so that the entire crop will die all at once so they can harvest immediately instead of waiting until the crops die and dry out naturally in waves.

Surely you have seen and heard the constant class-action lawsuit commercials against Monsanto for their Roundup product but Monsanto is another example of a major corporation that has knowingly poisoned, killed and injured untold numbers of people around the world. They pay a pathetic settlement and continue operating under governmental protections as always. See Chart 4 for more Monsanto companies.

Chart 3 – Monsanto-Owned Food Companies

Monsanto Companies DO NOT BUY	Hellmans	Ocean Spray
	Hershey's Nestle	Ore-Ida
	Holsum	Orville Redenbacher
Aunt Jemina	Hormel	Pasta-Roni
Aurora Foods	Hungry Jack	Pepperidge Farms
Banquet	Hunts	Pepsi
Best Foods	Interstate Bakeries	Pillsburry
Betty Crocker	Jiffy	Pop Secret
Bisquick	KC Masterpiece	Post Cereals
Cadburry	Keebler/Flowers Industries	Power Bar Brand
Campbells	Kelloggs	Prego Pasta Sauce
Capri Sun	Kid Cuisine	Pringles
Carnation	Knorr	Procter and Gamble
Chef Boyardee	Kool-Aid	Quaker
Coca Cola	Kraft/Phillip Morris	Ragu Sauce
ConAgra	Lean Cuisine	Rice-A-Roni
Delicious Brand Cookies	Lipton	Smart Ones
Duncan Hines	Loma Linda	Stouffers
Famous Amos	Marie Callenders	Sweppes
Frito Lay	Minute Made	Tombstone Pizza
General Mills	Morningstar	Totinos
Green Giant	Ms. Butterworths	Uncle Ben's
Healthy Choice	Nabisco	Unilever
Heinz	Nature Valley	V8

(Source:
www.i.pinimg.com/originals/93/9e/49/939e492b01f9151f2b2ccccf514f38b7.jp)

Chart 4 – Other Monsanto Companies

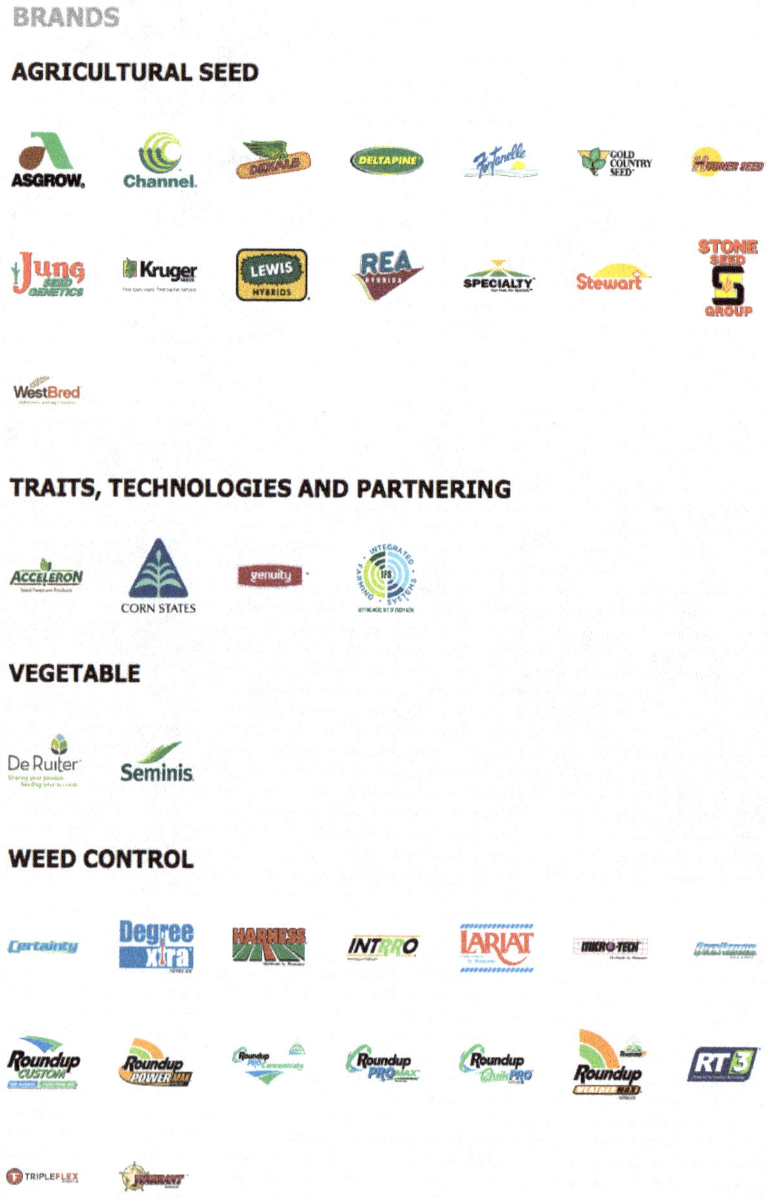

BRANDS

AGRICULTURAL SEED

ASGROW.   Channel.   DEKALB   DELTAPINE   Fontanelle   GOLD COUNTRY SEED   HUBNER SEED

Jung SEED GENETICS   Kruger   LEWIS HYBRIDS   REA HYBRIDS   SPECIALTY   Stewart   STONE SEED GROUP

WestBred

TRAITS, TECHNOLOGIES AND PARTNERING

ACCELERON   CORN STATES   genuity   INTEGRATED FARMING SYSTEMS

VEGETABLE

De Ruiter   Seminis

WEED CONTROL

Certainty   Degree Xtra   HARNESS   INTRRO   LARIAT   MICRO-TECH

Roundup CUSTOM   Roundup POWERMAX   Roundup PROConcentrate   Roundup PROMax   Roundup QuikPRO   Roundup WEATHER MAX   RT3

TRIPLEFLEX   WARRANT

(Source: www.seekingalpha.com/article/2378705-monsanto-international-seeds-of-growth)

PESKY PESTICIDE PROBLEMS

Below, see a list of pesticides that are in use in the United States. A great many of these are banned around the globe but are still unabashedly used in the US. Countless serious injury and death settlements have come from lawsuits pertaining to these toxic poisons that pose such serious health problems. Most are carcinogens and cause a vast spectrum of illnesses.

Pesticide	List	EU	USA	BRA	CHN
2,4-DB		3	3	1	1
Bensulide		1	3	1	0
Chloropicrin		1	3	0	2
Dichlobenil		1	3	1	4
Dicrotophos	W	1	3	1	0
EPTC		1	3	1	0
Norflurazon		1	3	1	0
Oxytetracycline	A	1	3	1	4
Paraquat	R2	1	3	2	1
Phorate	W, R2	1	3	1	2
Streptomycin	A	1	3	1	3
Terbufos	W	1	3	3	1
Tribufos (DEF)		1	3	1	0

Donley, Nathan. (2019). The USA lags behind other agricultural nations in banning harmful pesticides. Environmental Health. 18. 44. 10.1186/s12940-019-0488-0.

For reference, Red = banned/phasing out; Green = approved; Orange = Not approved/unknown

If you go down the list, you can see some familiar names. For instance, 2,4-D was half the formulation of Agent Orange, which was used as a chemical defoliant during the Vietnam era. 2,4-D has been linked to these illnesses according to the Veterans Affairs:

> If you served in Vietnam and have certain health conditions, VA presumes that these conditions are related to exposure to Agent Orange or other herbicides. VA presumes that the following health problems are related to herbicide exposure:
>
> - AL Amyloidosis
> - Chronic B-cell Leukemias
> - Chloracne
> - Diabetes Mellitus Type 2
> - Hodgkin's Disease
> - Ischemic Heart Disease
> - Multiple Myeloma
> - Non-Hodgkin's Lymphoma
> - Parkinson's Disease
> - Peripheral Neuropathy, Early- Onset
> - Porphyria Cutanea Tarda
> - Prostate Cancer
> - Respiratory Cancers
> - Soft Tissue Sarcomas
>
> In addition, VA presumes certain birth defects in children of Vietnam and Korea Veterans are associated with Veterans' qualifying military service.
>
> VA has recognized that certain birth defects among Veterans' children are associated with Veterans' qualifying service in Vietnam or Korea.
>
> - Spina bifida (except spina bifida occulta), a defect in the developing fetus that results in incomplete closing of the spine, is associated with Veterans' exposure to Agent Orange or other herbicides during qualifying service in Vietnam or Korea.
> - Birth defects in children of women Veterans is

associated with their military service in Vietnam but are not related to herbicide exposure.

Birth defects are abnormalities present at birth that result in mental or physical disabilities.

VA recognizes a wide range of birth defects as associated with women Veterans' service in Vietnam. These diseases are not tied to herbicides, including Agent Orange, or dioxin exposure, but rather to the birth mother's service in Vietnam.

Covered birth defects include, **but are not limited to**, the following conditions:

- o   Achondroplasia
- o   Cleft lip and cleft palate
- o   Congenital heart disease
- o   Congenital talipes equinovarus (clubfoot)
- o   Esophageal and intestinal atresia
- o   Hallerman-Streiff syndrome
- o   Hip dysplasia
- o   Hirschsprung's disease (congenital megacolon)
- o   Hydrocephalus due to aqueductal stenosis
- o   Hypospadias
- o   Imperforate anus
- o   Neural tube defects
- o   Poland syndrome
- o   Pyloric stenosis
- o   Syndactyly (fused digits)
- o   Tracheoesophageal fistula
- o   Undescended testicle
- o   Williams syndrome

(Source: www.publichealth.va.gov)

If this is the damage just *one* of these chemicals can do, what do they do in concert with the other chemical toxins and engineered foods?

PESTICIDES: BUT WAIT, THERE'S MORE!

We cannot explore all of these poisons in this book, but we will take a look at a couple more, such as Paraquat (paraquat dichloride). This herbicide comes in several brands such as Gramoxone, Helmquat, Firestorm, Parazone and others. According to the EPA, paraquat is so harmful to humans that "one sip can kill." There is no antidote for poisoning from paraquat ingestion.

Paraquat mixes easily in food, water or other beverages. To prevent accidental ingestion, paraquat contains "safeguard additives" such as dyes, vomiting agents and odors.

Small amounts of paraquat can cause:

- Lung scarring
- Heart failure
- Liver failure
- Kidney failure

Large amounts of paraquat can cause:

- Liver failure
- Coma
- Confusion
- Acute kidney failure
- Fast heart rate
- Heart injury
- Muscle weakness
- Fluid in the lungs
- Respiratory failure that may lead to death
- Seizures
- Scarring of the lungs
- Death

PARAQUAT & PARKINSON'S

Studies have linked paraquat exposure to Parkinson's Disease. Estimates of the risk vary depending on the study but in one 2011 study by Caroline M. Tanner and colleagues, published in Environmental Health Perspectives, researchers found study participants with Parkinson's were 2.5 times more likely to have used paraquat or another herbicide called rotenone.

The New York Times reported paraquat can increase the risk of Parkinson's by 150 percent.

The Michael J. Fox Foundation for Parkinson's Research cites that people exposed to paraquat at a young age had a 200 to 600 percent increased risk of developing Parkinson's.

The link between the herbicide and Parkinson's disease has led to a growing number of paraquat lawsuits against the weedkiller's manufacturers.

(Source: www.consumernotice.org)

DON'T FORGET ROUNDUP!

To conclude this section, we must look at Roundup, manufactured by Monsanto and later bought out by Bayer. Roundup is one of the most used pesticides in every aspect of agriculture, household and commercial industries—you probably have a jug in your garage now. Monsanto even makes GMO seeds that are touted as "Roundup Ready" seeds that are resistant to Roundup. The massive amounts of Roundup used are compounded each year as more and more weeds are growing tolerant of it. The next pages contain charts with Roundup usage per state and by year. Roundup has had a slew of legal battles but is still probably the most widely used out of the group—showing Monsanto is as resistant to decimation as its GMO products.

Monsanto has settled over 100,000 Roundup lawsuits, paying out about $11 billion as of May 2022. There are still 30,000 lawsuits pending. This includes 4,000 cases in multidistrict litigation (MDL) in California. MDL cases are not class-action suits. Instead they group cases together so that instead of answering the same question repeatedly in each separate lawsuit, the courts can resolve some specific issues for all of them at once.

In June 2022, the Ninth Circuit filed a decision in a Roundup case. In the court's opinion, the Ninth Circuit urged the Environmental Protection Agency (EPA) to reconsider its conclusion that Roundup does not cause substantial harm to people or the environment. Also in that month, the Supreme Court dismissed an appeal by Bayer in another Roundup case.

In July 2022, the 11th Circuit ruled that Bayer had failed to adequately warn about the risk of cancer from Roundup.

While the EPA suggests that there's no direct link, the International Agency for Research on Cancer's stance is more in line with scientific evidence. A study from the University of Washington found that exposure to glyphosate increased an individual's risk of non-Hodgkin's lymphoma by 41%. That is significant.

The CDC recently released findings that up to 80% of Americans may have traces of Roundup in their urine, showing they have been exposed to it. Considering that 200 million pounds of Roundup are sprayed annually on U.S. crops, it is not surprising most of the population has been exposed to it.

If you have used Roundup even once, you could be at a higher risk of cancer. See your doctor regularly to watch out for symptoms."

(Source: www.forbes.com/advisor/legal/product-liability/roundup-lawsuit-

update/)

We have only briefly looked at three of these deadly chemicals that are applied to our food, our cotton and the feed that livestock consume. As of now there are still two hundred forty-one more chemicals (pesticide, herbicide, fungicide, etc.) we could explore, each one having their own unique history of destruction, and almost all are carcinogens.

Finally, we have only looked at one producer of these chemicals & GMO's; there are many more. We all, at some point, have at least trace amounts of these chemicals in our food and bodies along with other contaminants that are present in our food, water and other products such as mercury, arsenic, lead, cadmium, dioxins and PCB's. But wait, there's more!

- 6 -

GMO's: CHRONIC ILLNESS & INFLAMMATION

It is my opinion that Bt-infused GMO's are the catalyst for many major diseases, chronic illness, auto immune disease and allergies (all of which are a form of inflammation). Genetically modified organisms are a perversion of the original creation and they are an abomination—they have been called "Frankenfoods" for good reason. The FDA claims they are no different than naturally hybrid plants, which have been produced since agriculture began. This is far from the truth as there is no way completely separate organisms can do this under natural circumstances—plants do not breed with animals.

What these "scientists" are doing is taking genes from one species and forcing them into a completely different organism. We already discussed the Bt bacteria that has now had its genes forced into corn, tomato, potato, eggplant, soy and cotton. Another example would be GMO/GE (Genetically Engineered) salmon that was developed by AquaBounty Technologies Inc. This company splices growth genes from a Chinook salmon and a seal eel onto an Atlantic salmon, which then enables that fish to grow twice as fast as a regular Atlantic salmon. Salmon is also modified genetically with salmon lice to make them more resistant to salmon lice infestation. But what are the long-term consequences and ramifications for these extra-natural procedures?

For more on this topic, look for an excellent research paper called

"Genetically Engineered Crops, Glyphosate and the Deterioration of Health in the United States" by Nancy L. Swanson, Andre Leu, Jon Abrahamson and Bradley Wallett.

(Source: people.csail.mit.edu/seneff/Swanson_et_al_2014.pdf)

In the next few pages there will be many charts that show a pattern between GMO crops, glyphosate use and illness that are taken from the aforementioned study. The only thing this report was missing was the definition of what is the exact cause of all the illness. Keep in mind that Bt-laced GMO crops are the cause of leaky gut and the primary catalyst for all these conditions, as I have explained in previous chapters. With leaky gut, your intestines become porous so toxins such as raw food, pesticides and heavy metals can directly enter the blood stream, causing an autoimmune reaction, chronic inflammation, malnutrition and allowing more toxins to be absorbed than what would occur from a random exposure event. Keep this in mind as you examine the graphs from the study.

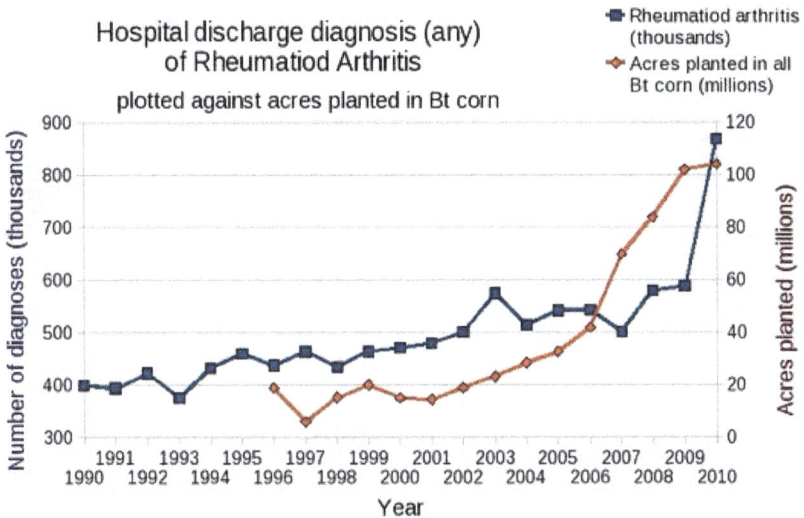

(Source: people.csail.mit.edu/seneff/Swanson_et_al_2014.pdf)

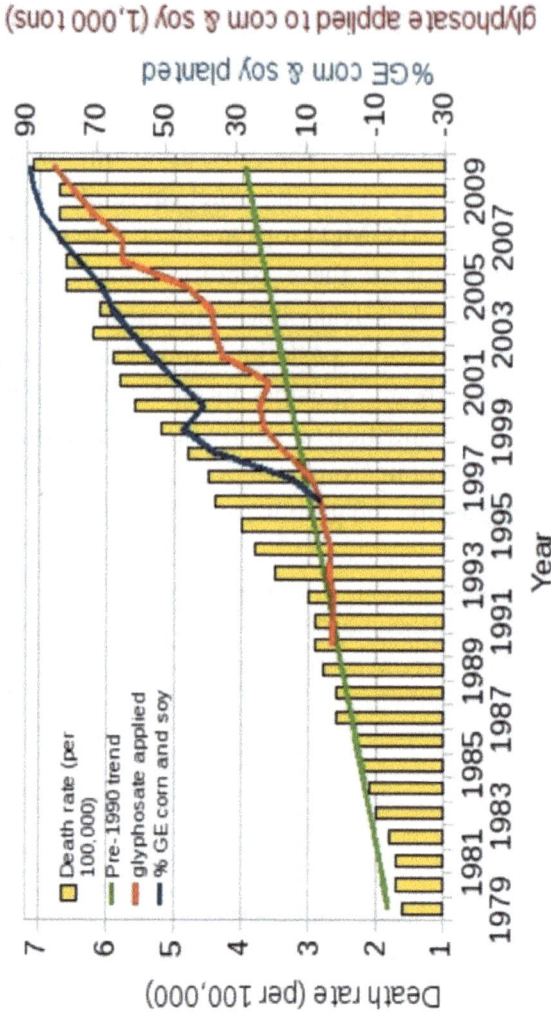

Figure 25. Correlation between Parkinson's disease deaths and glyphosate use & GE crop growth.

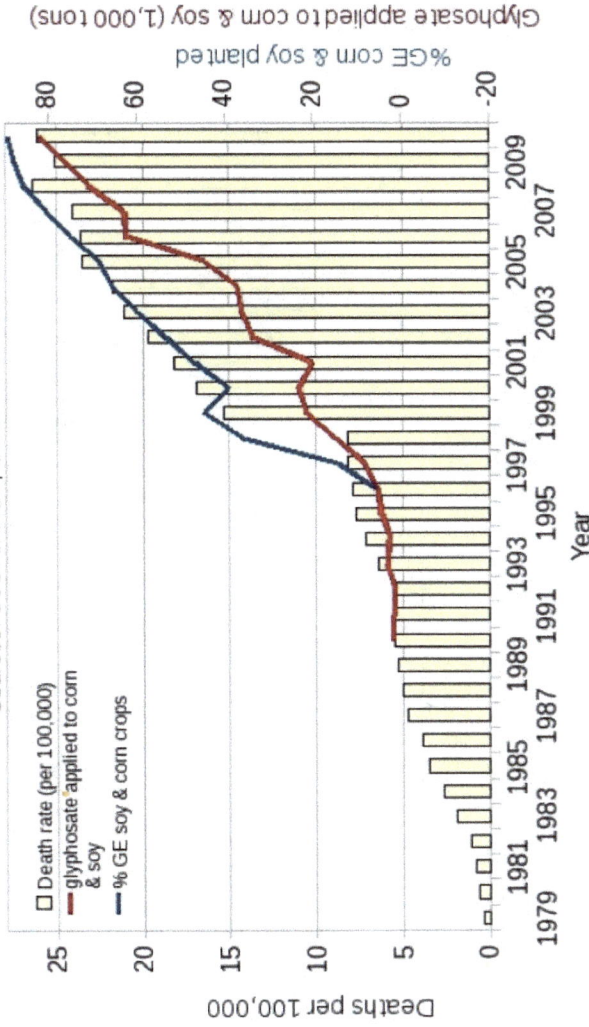

Figure 26. Correlation between Alzheimer's disease deaths and glyphosate use & GE crop growth.

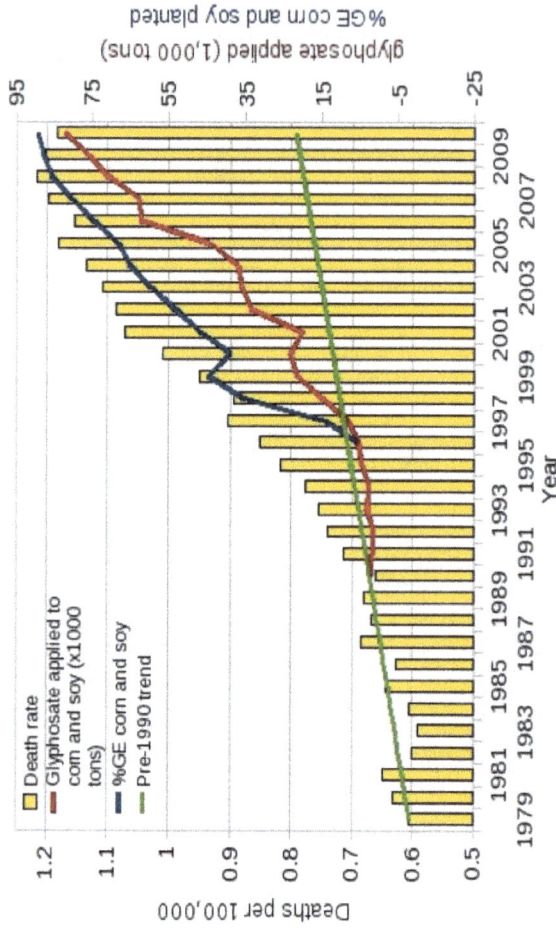

Deaths due to Multiple Sclerosis (ICD G35 & 340)
plotted against percentage of GE soy & corn (R = 0.9477, p <= 6.339e-06) and glyphosate applied to soy & corn (R = 0.9005, p <= 5.079e-07) sources: USDA:NASS; CDC

Figure 24. Correlation between multiple sclerosis deaths and glyphosate use & GE crop growth.

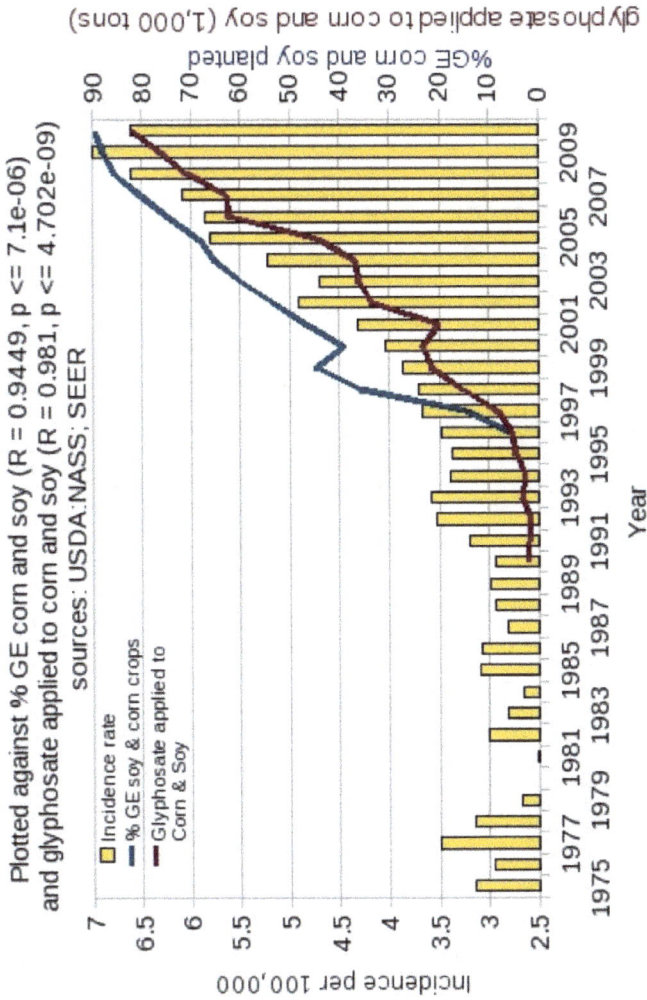

Figure 8. Correlation between bladder/urinary tract cancer and glyphosate use & GE crop growth.

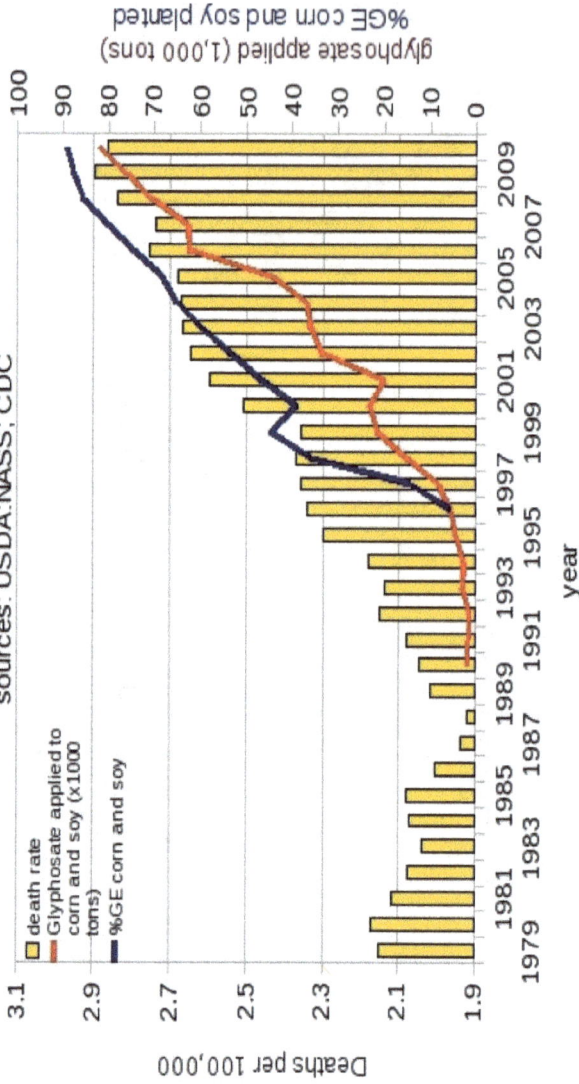

Figure 12. Correlation between myeloid leukaemia deaths and glyphosate use & GE crop growth.

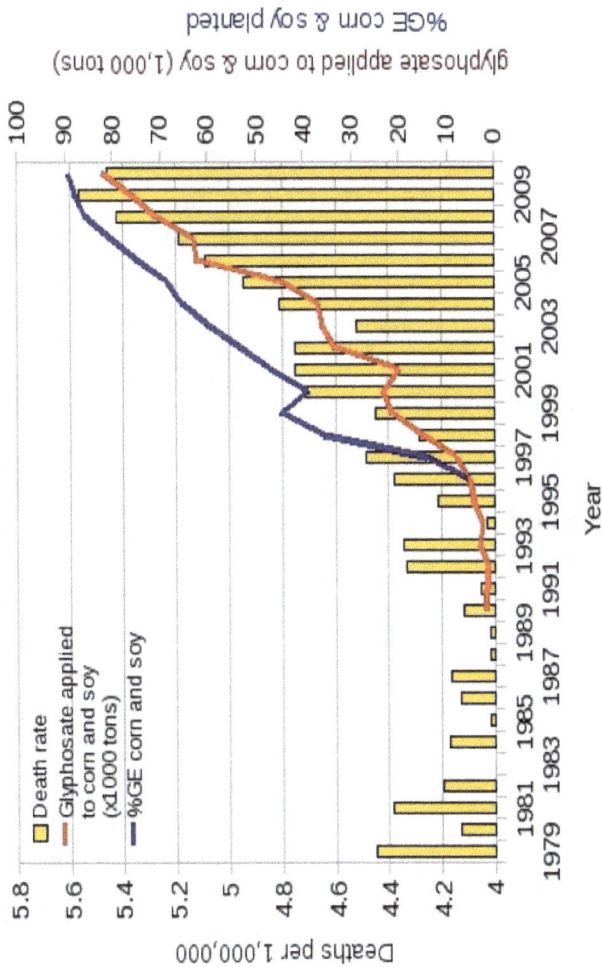

Figure 10. Correlation between thyroid cancer deaths and glyphosate use & GE crop growth.

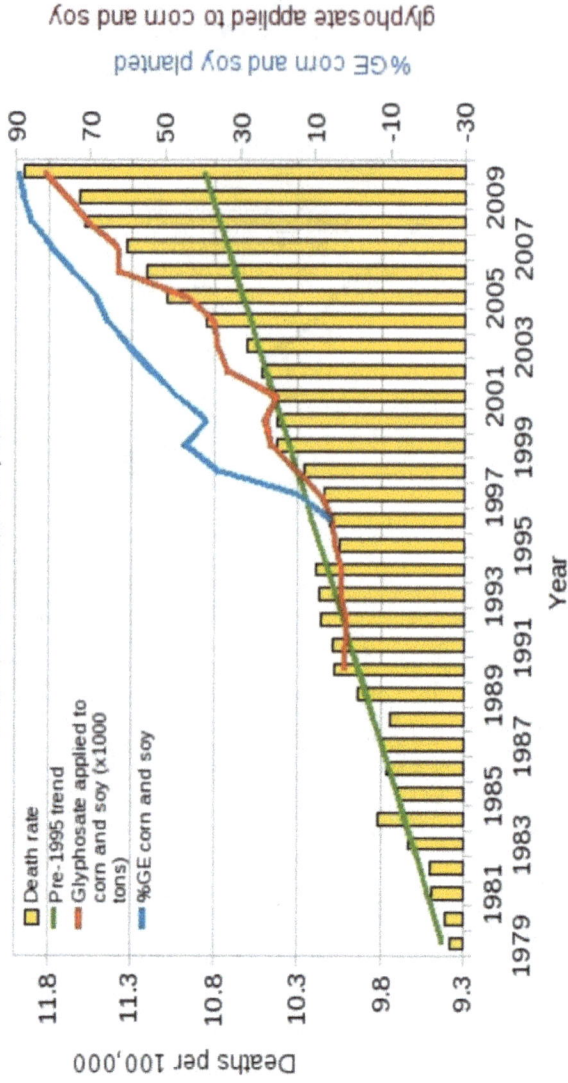

Figure 13. Correlation between pancreatic cancer deaths and glyphosate use & GE crop growth.

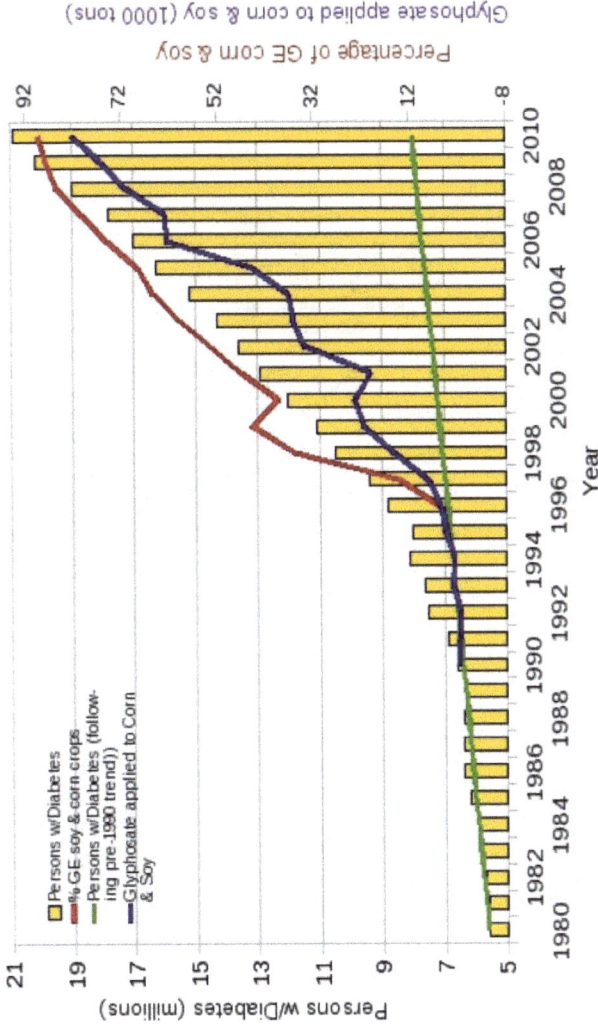

Figure 18. Correlation between diabetes prevalence and glyphosate use & GE crop growth.

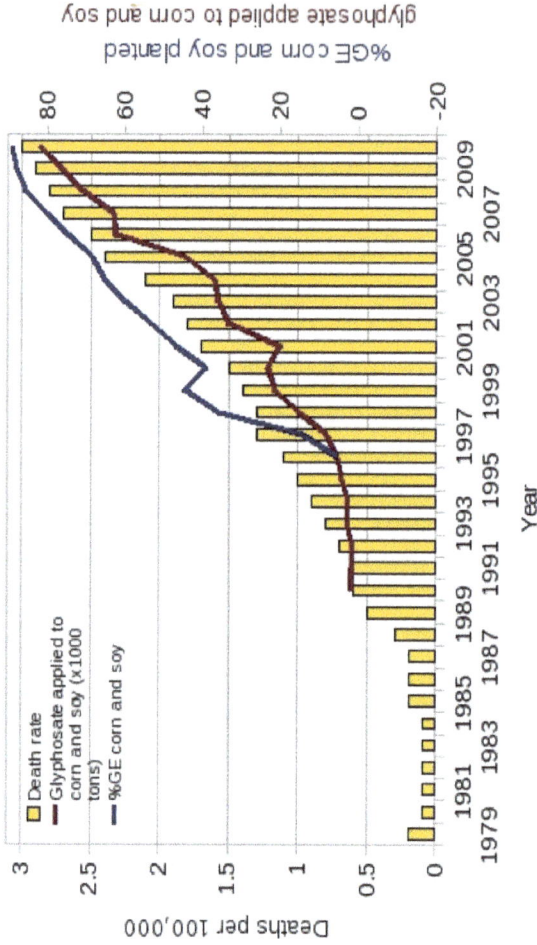

Deaths due to Disorders of Lipoprotein Metabolism
(ICD E78.5 hyperlipoproteinemia & E78.0 hypercholesterolemia)

plotted against %GE corn & soy (R = 0.9554, p <= 4.597e-06)
and glyphosate applied to corn & soy (R = 0.9775, p <= 5.941e-09)
sources: USDA:NASS; CDC

Figure 19. Correlation between lipoprotein disorder deaths and glyphosate use & GE crop growth. Hyperlipoproteinemia is the largest contribution to the deaths.

70

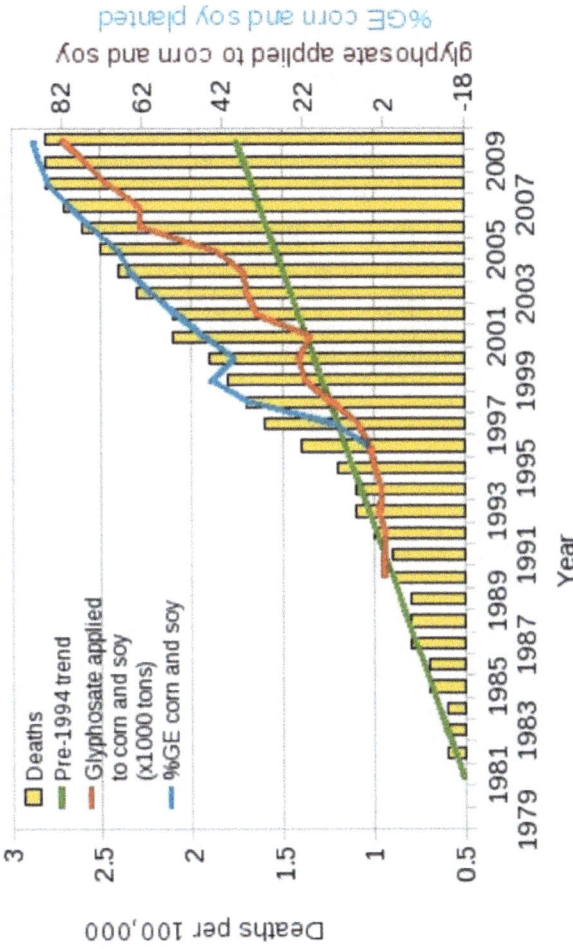

Figure 15. Correlation between stroke deaths and glyphosate use & GE crop growth.

(Charts on pages 62-71 all from
people.csail.mit.edu/seneff/Swanson_et_al_2014.pdf)

As you can see from the charts, there is a sharp rise in almost all of these chronic illnesses and inflammations beginning in 1994, the same year Bt-laced GMO crops became available in supermarkets. We have seen this same sharp rise in allergies from the previous chapter on GMO's. There is a definitive correlation between the hypertrophic outbreak of allergies, chronic illness, autism, chronic inflammation and the introduction of GMO's. We must rally together, educate each other and petition our leadership to abolish this abomination. One of our biggest weapons is to say it with cash—stop buying their poison and they will change but be wary of rebranded or new products as well!

- 7 -

THE DANGERS OF FOOD ADDITIVES

Artificial food additives can be classified as preservatives, sweeteners, colors, flavors, spices, flavor enhancers, fat replacers, nutrients, emulsifiers, stabilizers, thickeners, binders, texturizers, pH control, acidulants, leavening agents, anti-caking agents, yeast nutrients, dough conditioners, dough strengtheners, firming agents, enzyme preparations, gasses, anti-foaming agents and other deceptive labels. These additives are made from petroleum, GMO corn, metals, GMO soy and other problematic substances.

FOOD COLORINGS

Basically all of the synthetic colorings or dyes used in food in the US are problematic. Natural colorants from berries, beets, spirulina, annatto, etc. are already food so they are excellent substitutes. The following list shows the problematic coloring sources that are in almost everything we eat—from food to medicines and supplements.

Many food dyes have been delisted for a variety of reasons, ranging from poor coloring properties to regulatory restrictions. Many used in the US are banned in the EU and other countries. We will explore the reasons some have been banned and then we will move to health concerns of currently approved food dyes.

Dye/Colorant	Associated Health Issues	Banned?
Red No. 2	Carcinogenic	Yes
Red No. 4	Carcinogenic	Yes
Red No. 32	Carcinogenic, genotoxic	Yes
Orange No. 1	Carcinogenic, genotoxic	Yes
Orange No. 2	Carcinogenic, genotoxic	Yes
Yellow No. 1-4	Carcinogenic	Yes
Violet No. 1	None listed but terminated from use	Yes
Blue No. 1	Causes kidney tumors in lab mice	No
Blue No. 2	Increases tumor risks, especially in brain	No
Green No. 3	Increased tumors in testes and bladders of lab rats	No
Red No. 3	Thyroid carcinogen	No
Red No. 40	Allergic reactions, ADHD hyperactivity in children, accelerates tumors in mice	No
Yellow No. 5	Hypersensitivity, hyperactivity disorders and behavior problems in children	No
Yellow No. 6	Hypersensitivity and severe hyperactivity in children; linked to adrenal tumors	No
Titanium Dioxide	Carcinogenic; lung, brain, kidney, other organ damage; inflammatory bowel disease	No
Caramel Color	Under multiple other nomenclatures; digestive issues, obesity, weight gain, malnutrition, heart disease, diabetes, cancer, leaky gut, etc.	No

(Source: www.en.wikipedia.org/wiki/Food_coloring)

With the history of artificial food coloring in this country and the current trends, please give careful consideration before consuming or handing your children any products containing these dyes. They are found in most mainstream foods, cosmetics, pet food and pharmaceuticals. Almost everything that is marketed to children is brightly colored with these artificial dyes and loaded with other dangerous ingredients.

FOOD PRESERVATIVES

The next in the list of dangerous ingredients is food preservatives. Some are labeled as "antioxidants" and as "synthetic vitamin E" (tocopherols) so do not be deceived, they are not there for your benefit, just for the "illusion of health."

Helpful Hint: To know whether you are looking at a natural or a synthetic substance, look at the ending. If it ends with an "-ide" or "-ate" it is a synthetic salt version. This is true for vitamin supplements as well.

The following is from the FDA approved food preservatives list. We will look at the most problematic on this list.

- **Sodium Benzoate**
  - ALSO: *a synthetic chemical; other names: Benzoic acid sodium salt, phenylcarboxylic acid sodium salt, Benzenecarboxylic acid sodium salt, dracylic acid sodium salt, E211 and others*
  - converts easily to benzene, a known carcinogen.
  - exposure to heat, light and long storage increase benzene conversion
  - it can cause nausea, abdominal pain, and vomiting
  - it will deplete amino acid levels needed for energy production
  - is known to cause inflammation, oxidative stress, allergies, ADHD, and upset appetite control
  - it could also be contributing to cancer and hyperactivity

- **Potassium Bromate**
  - a possible human carcinogen added to the flour of many packaged baked goods
  - in animal studies, causes kidney and thyroid cancers
  - is banned in several countries, including Brazil, Canada, the European Union and the United Kingdom
- **Propylparaben Sodium**
  - ALSO: *Sodium Salt of E216, sodium salt of Propylparaben, Propylparaben sodium, E217, Propyl-P-Hydroxybenzoate Sodium Salt*
  - as a paraben, potential harms can include infertility, developmental issues, cancer, violently allergic reactions, hormonal disruption and more
- **Propylparaben**
  - ALSO: *Solbrol P, Nipasol, E216, Propyl-P-Hydroxybenzoate*
  - as a paraben, it can cause cancer, fertility problems, developmental issues, hormonal disruption, violent allergic reactions and more.
- **TBHQ**
  - ALSO: *Tertiary Butylhydroquinone, 2-tert-Butyl-1,4-benzenediol, Avox BHT-T, Butylhydroxinon, E319, Tert-Butylhydroquinone*
  - it likely has a profound negative impact on the immune system and immune response
  - other side effects may include vomiting, ringing in the ears, nausea; convulsions and visual disturbances are also possible
  - any amount can lead to stomach tumors and DNA damage
- **Brominated Vegetable Oil or BVO**
  - brominated compounds have been linked to numerous health hazards, including harm to the nervous system

- o BVO can build up in the body and research has shown a connection between drinking large amounts of BVO-containing sodas over a long period and problems such as headaches, irritation of the skin and mucous membranes, fatigue and loss of muscle coordination, memory problems, reproductive health issues and more
- o BVO has been banned in many countries

- **Erythorbic Acid**
  - o ALSO: *Isoascorbic Acid, D-Araboascorbic Acid, Threo-Ascorbic Acid, Erythorbic Acid Anhydride, Erythroascorbic Acid, Erythorbic Acid Lactone, Saccharosonic Acid, E315, Erythorbic Acid*
  - o it can cause headaches, fatigue, hemolysis, dizziness and body flushing
  - o upset stomach, diarrhea and other gastrointestinal issues are possible
  - o it can cause inaccurate blood glucose tests
  - o it can trigger kidney stones and gout symptoms in people with past diseases

- **Sodium Nitrite**
  - o nitrites can form nitrosamines, which are cancer-causing compounds
  - o impairs oxygen transport, increased risk of stomach cancer, type 1 diabetes and possibly linked to Alzheimer's Disease

- **Calcium Sorbate**
  - o synthetic substance, likely harmful
  - o banned in the EU

- **Potassium Sorbate**
  - o synthetic substance shown in studies to damage white blood cells, which damages gene information, which can lead to cancer, DNA damage and other disease
  - o can cause nausea, diarrhea, migraines, nutrient loss from foods, reproductive toxicity, developmental

toxicity, allergies, genotoxicity and other hazards.

- **BHA**
  - ALSO: *n-Butylated Hydroxyanisole, Butylhydroxyanisole, Tert-butyl-4-methoxyphenol, Antioxidant 29, 3-tert-butyl-4-hydroxyanisole, 2(3)-tert-Butyl-4-hydroxyanisole, Antioxidant BHA, E320, Butylated Hydroxyanisole*
  - immunotoxic effect can increase susceptibility to autoimmune diseases and infections
  - this additive can also cause liver damage, bring about developmental and reproductive toxicity, disrupt hormone balance and possibly even induce cancer
  - can cause elevated cholesterol levels, insomnia, hyperactivity, urticaria and asthma
  - possible allergic reactions
  - in combination with vitamin C, it can induce free radicals and damage DNA
- **BHT**
  - ALSO: *Dibutylhydroxytoluene, Butylhydroxytoluene, Agidol, Tert-Butyl-4-Hydroxytoluene, DBPC (Di-Tert-Butylphenol), 2,6-Di-Tert-Butyl-4-Methylphenol, Butylated Hydroxyanisole, Sustane BHT, Vanox B, Antrancine 8, Advastab 401, E321, Butylated Hydroxytoluene and others*
  - it can cause migraines and liver damage
  - there are cancer-inducing dangers associated with it
  - is known to cause mutagenic changes in humans
  - it can have negative hormonal effects, cause skin irritation, asthma, as well as various allergic reactions such as difficulty breathing, hives and itching
- **EDTA**
  - ALSO: *calcium disodium EDTA (ethylene-diaminetetraacetate*

o researchers hypothesize that EDTA may disrupt the intestinal barrier and increase intestinal permeability, so people with inflammatory bowel diseases may especially want to avoid

(Source: www.yourhealthremedy.com)

ANTI-FOAMING AGENTS

Antifoaming agents are another fun additive that saves corporations money and hassle at the expense of your health.

- **Dimethylpolysiloxane**
  - o ALSO: *polydimethylsiloxane*
  - o a toxic industrial chemical that is partially derived from silicone
  - o characterized by its vinegar-like odor and is traditionally used in the manufacturing of various *commercial* products such as silicone lubricants, polishes and grease, bathroom caulk or sealants, defoaming agents and cosmetic products
  - o the silicone derivative is also commonly found in heat transfer fluids, aquarium sealant and kinetic sand as well as silly putty and even breast implants
  - o causes cataract, hypotony and corneal abrasion, triggers acute pneumonitis and acute respiratory distress syndrome
  - o exposure may also result in diffuse alveolar hemorrhage, fever and hypoxia
  - o raises the odds of dyspnea, altered mental status and blood-stained mucus
  - o causes skin irritations, nausea, vomiting and diarrhea, as well as being especially harmful to both the skin and the digestive system

(Source: www.fda.gov/food/food-additives-and-gras-ingredients-information-consumers/types-food-ingredients)

NOT SO SWEET SWEETENERS

- **Sugar/cane sugar:** consuming high amounts of raw cane sugar can contribute to weight gain and may promote the development of chronic conditions like heart disease and diabetes
- **Sorbitol:** consuming high amounts of sorbitol can cause digestive issues such as bloating, gas, stomach pain, cramps and diarrhea, especially for people with IBS
- **High Fructose Corn Syrup:** linked to many serious health issues, including diabetes, obesity and heart disease, as well as potential toxins from being a GMO product.
- **Saccharin:** can lead to alterations in the gut microbiome and may reduce good gut bacteria, which play a central role in everything from immune function to digestive health. Disruptions in the beneficial bacteria in your gut may also be linked to health issues, including obesity, inflammatory bowel disease (IBD) and colorectal cancer
- **Aspartame**
  - ALSO: *N-(L-α-Aspartyl)-L-phenylalanine-1-methyl ester, APM, Aspartyl phenylalanine methyl ester, Splenda, NutraSweet, Equal, AminoSweet, Sweet'N Low, Canderel*
  - Extremely harmful substance with high likelihood of causing depression, cancer, brain damage, weight gain, obesity, diabetes, cardiovascular disease, dementia, Alzheimer's, stroke, mood disorders, seizures, headaches, migraines, metabolic issues, kidney damage, anxiety, learning problems, digestive issues, fertility problems, liver damage, and even pre-term birth and overweight babies
- **Sucralose:** consuming sucralose increases blood sugar and insulin levels, may be linked to reductions in good gut bacteria, causes a higher risk of inflammation and increased weight gain. Baking with sucralose can also be dangerous due to the formation of chloropropanols, which are chemical

compounds thought to be toxic.

- **Acesulfame Potassium**: causes impaired mental function and memory. Possible carcinogen, increased weight gain in male animals and negatively altered gut bacteria in both sexes during animal testing.
- **Neotame:** is chemically similar to aspartame, which is widely regarded as the most dangerous artificial sweetener. Both neotame and aspartame convert to formaldehyde when metabolized. However, the effects of neotame may be even worse because it includes 3-dimethylbutyl—one of the world's most hazardous chemicals, according to the Environmental Protection Agency (EPA).
- **Erythritol:** in combination with aspartame may produce anxiety, fibromyalgia, fatigue, memory loss, weight gain and possibly more.
- **Xylitol:** (Erythritol, Maltitol, Mannitol, Sorbitol and other sugar alcohols that end in "–itol".) Additionally, it has gastrointestinal side effects that include bloating, gas, cramping and diarrhea. Its laxative effect is so pronounced that it is actually part of the chemical makeup for many over-the-counter laxatives.

(Source: www.fda.gov/food/food-additives-and-gras-ingredients-information-consumers/types-food-ingredients)

Even though these sweeteners have been on the market for decades, pregnant and breastfeeding women should select a natural sweetener instead. WebMD states: "Not enough is known about the use of xylitol during pregnancy and breast feeding. Stay on the safe side and avoid use."

Source: https://www.webmd.com/drugs/2/drug-154371/sodium-fluoride-with-xylitol-oral/details

Special note to dog owners: Sugar alcohol-based artificial sweeteners are a life-threatening toxin to dogs. Be mindful of breath mints, candies, sugar-free gum, frozen desserts and other foods containing these sweeteners when your pets are around.

OTHER ADDITIVES

Spices

Many spices test positive for heavy metals (lead, mercury, cadmium, arsenic) so checking consumer report websites is suggested. The most common spices that test positive are paprika, oregano, turmeric, ginger, basil, cumin, thyme. McCormick brand spices tend to have the worst ratings so do your research.

(Source: consumerreports.org/health/food-safety/your-herbs-and-spices-might-
contain-arsenic-cadmium-and-lead-a6246621494/)

Candy

Cadmium and lead have been found in dark chocolate. High levels of lead have been found in many candies from Mexico and China, most come from candies containing tamarindo and chili.

Flavor Enhancers

- **Monosodium glutamate (MSG)** has been associated with an increased risk of metabolic disorders, primarily based on animal studies that have linked the additive to insulin resistance, high blood sugar levels and diabetes. Some studies claim that MSG can lead to brain toxicity by causing excessive glutamate levels in the brain that overstimulate nerve cells, resulting in cell death. MSG allergies can cause weakness, flushing, dizziness, headache, numbness, muscle tightness, difficulty breathing and even the loss of consciousness. Colloquially, there are wide anecdotal reports of Chinese Restaurant Syndrome—the numbness of the neck, arms and back with headache, dizziness, and palpitations, often mimicking a heart attack.
- **Hydrolyzed soy protein** can cause mild forms of a soy allergy, resulting in hives, swelling, tingling or itching in the mouth. Some people may also experience redness of the skin, diarrhea, nausea and vomiting.
- **Autolyzed yeast extract** can cause mild flushing of the skin

82

as well as headaches
- **Disodium guanylate/inosinate**
  - ALSO: *sodium 5'-guanylate and disodium 5'-guanylate, Sodium 5'-inosinate, Disodium inosin 5'-monophosphate, Inosine 5', disodium phosphate, Sodium inosinate*
  - People who are sensitive to MSG may want to avoid disodium glutamate/inosinate, as these additives are often paired together.
  - Those with gout or a history of uric acid kidney stones should also avoid disodium guanylate. Guanylates often metabolize to purines, which are compounds that can raise uric acid levels in your body.

(Source: https://www.mayoclinic.org/healthy-lifestyle/nutrition-and-healthy-eating/expert-answers/monosodium-glutamate/faq-20058196)

Fat Replacers

- **Olestra (Olean)** can cause diarrhea and loose stools, abdominal cramps, flatulence and other adverse effects, sometimes severely. Olestra reduces the body's ability to absorb fat-soluble carotenoids (such as alpha and beta-carotene, lycopene, lutein and canthaxanthin) from fruits and vegetables.
- **Carrageenan** may promote or cause inflammation, irritable bowel syndrome, bloating, glucose intolerance, colon cancer and food allergies. Increased inflammation can cause inflammatory bowel disease, arthritis, chronic cholecystitis or gall bladder inflammation.
- **Polydextrose** in large quantities, or in particularly sensitive people, can cause a variety of side effects including abdominal cramping, bloating, diarrhea and excessive gas.

Nutrients

"Nutrients" are vitamins and minerals added to replace those lost during the manufacturing process. Most or all are synthetic and some are not naturally occurring in our food sources (such as ferrous sulfate, which is an inorganic iron that destroys vitamin E). A good deal of food additives come from GMO corn and soy. The most common nutrients added to foods are:

- thiamine hydrochloride
- riboflavin (Vitamin B$_2$)
- niacin, niacinamide
- folate or folic acid
- beta carotene
- potassium iodide
- iron or ferrous sulfate
- alpha tocopherols
- ascorbic acid
- vitamin D
- amino acids
  - L-tryptophan
  - L-lysine
  - L-leucine
  - L-methionine

Emulsifiers

These additives allow for smooth mixing of ingredients and prevent product separation.

- **Soy lecithin** in high amounts, can cause diarrhea, bloating, stomach upset and other digestive issues. A small percentage of people may experience an allergic reaction. Additionally, it may not serve us well when it comes to drug interactions with medications in the cholesterol-lowering and blood-thinning categories.

- **Polysorbates**
  - ALSO: *Polysorbate 20, Polysorbate 80, polyoxyethylene (20) sorbitan monolaurate, polyoxyethylene (80) sorbitan monooleate*
  - Polysorbate 80 links to various side effects, according to a 2018 study.
  - Small amounts of undigested polysorbate 80 in meals may promote bacterial translocation, explaining why Crohn's disease is becoming more common.
  - Polysorbate 80 also links to a variety of systemic responses such as hypersensitivity, non-allergic anaphylaxis and rash, and injection and infusion-site adverse effects in medication formulations (pain, erythema and thrombophlebitis).
- **Propylene glycol**
  - ALSO: *Methyl ethyl glycol, 1,2-dihydroxypropane, Trimethyl glycol, 1,2-propanediol*
  - Food additive that belongs to the same chemical group as alcohol.
  - Some studies claim it causes heart attacks, kidney and liver failure and brain problems; other studies say it is safe.
  - In the US it is considered GRAS (**g**enerally **r**ecognized **a**s **s**afe), it is restricted use in the EU.
  - If you have compromised kidney/liver function it can lead to a buildup of propylene glycol and lactic acid in the bloodstream, causing symptoms of toxicity.

PH Control & Acidulants

These additives control acidity, alkalinity and prevent spoilage of products.

- **Phosphoric acid**
  - ALSO: *orthophosphoric acid, monophosphoric acid, white phosphoric acid, phosphoric (V) acid, orthophosphoric acid mono-, di-, and tri-basic, food-*

grade phosphoric acid, thermal phosphoric acid and E338

- o In high amounts, it can contribute to cavities, dental erosion, kidney disease and osteoporosis.
- o It may also chip away at bone health, and indirectly contribute to weight gain and various metabolic disorders.
- o Being sensitive to it may cause gastrointestinal discomfort, acid reflux or heartburn. People with acid-related gastrointestinal disorders (such as GERD, gastritis, or peptic ulcer disease) and kidney disease should be careful when consuming it or simply avoid it completely.

- **Magnesium Phosphate**
  - o ALSO: *magnesium dihydrogen phosphate, acid magnesium phosphate, monobasic magnesium phosphate, magnesium hydrogen phosphate, magnesium phosphate monohydrate, and dibasic magnesium phosphate, magnesium hydrogen phosphate trihydrate, magnesium phosphate tribasic trihydrate, and magnesium orthophosphate trihydrate, Magnesium orthophosphate, Magnesium acid phosphate, Magnesium polyphosphate*
  - o Potential side effects in truly excessive amounts are pretty much the same as is the case with Calcium Phosphate.
  - o Can lead to diarrhea, stomach upset, kidney damage and electrolyte imbalances (cause mal-absorption of minerals like calcium, potassium and sodium).

- **Ammonium Hydroxide** is poisonous but very difficult to find information about ever since the "Pink Slime" meat information has come out; it would be best to avoid this until further studies have been done.
- **Trisodium Phosphate (TSP)** is irritating to the gastric

mucosa, likely binds important trace minerals, leading to malnutrition. Widely found in children's breakfast cereals. Notably the same chemical formula found in the cleaner TSP that is great for degreasing and removing mold and mildew.

Leavening Agents

These additives promote the rising of baked goods.

- **Baking Powder as Sodium Aluminum Sulfate** is a suspected risk factor in Alzheimer's disease and that aluminum directly influences the process of Alzheimer's disease.
- **Disodium pyrophosphate DSP**
  - ALSO: *Sodium Pyrophosphate, Sodium Hexametaphosphate, Sodium Tripolyphosphate, Sodium Dihydrogen Phosphate, Sodium Monohydrogen Phosphate, Sodium Phosphate Tribasic, Sodium Acid Phosphate, Tetrasodium Pyrophosphate, MSP, DSP, TSP, E339, Sodium Phosphate and others*
  - Sodium phosphate can prove to be problematic only when consumed in high amounts.
  - The most prominent issue is the fact that it can create profound electrolyte imbalances in minerals like calcium, magnesium and potassium.
  - This can negatively impact heart health, muscle function and bone health.
  - High amounts can also lead to kidney damage, abdominal pain and other digestive issues, and dehydration.
  - It can also interfere with medications for blood pressure and antibiotics.

Anti-Caking Agents

These keep food free-flowing and prevent moisture absorption.

- **Calcium silicate, calcium orthosilicate, or calcium silicon oxide** are inhalation hazards, and may possibly have similar effects as silicon dioxide (see below).
- **Iron ammonia citrate** ammonium ferric citrate, ferric ammonium citrate, ammonium iron (III) citrate can cause gastrointestinal disease, but information is difficult to access for research.
- **Silicon dioxide** is an oxide of silicon with the chemical formula SiO_2, most commonly found in nature as quartz.
  - It is in many foods to prevent caking and has been explored as a possible pesticide in microcrystalline and nanoparticulate size.
  - <u>**This is the problem with table salt**</u>, the salt itself is not the problem, it is the microcrystalline glass (silica) in it that is the problem. If you inhale silica, it causes respiratory issues from the tissues becoming micro-lacerated. The same thing happens in your bloodstream, causing the vessels to be micro-abraded so the body responds with cholesterol to repair itself. Check your table salt for silicon dioxide!
  - Use Himalayan salt or Real Salt from Utah. The concern with sea salt is the lack of nutrients and the possibility of all the poisons that are present in the ocean near the coasts (pesticides, heavy metals etc.).

Dough Conditioners

These chemicals are added to produce stable doughs. They include ammonium sulfate, polysorbate, ammonium chloride and potassium bromate, which we covered earlier. Additionally,

- **Azodicarbonamide** aka "Yoga Mat", azo(*bis*)formamide, ADA, ADCA
  - Contains semicarbazide, a known carcinogen, known to cause asthma and respiratory issues in exposed production workers and, when baked, caused cancer in lab mice.

- o Azodicarbonamide is synthesized from:
  - *Urea*: nitrogenic substance found in urine
  - *Hydrazine*: a toxic substance used in creating foams, agrochemicals, a propellant for spacecraft, automotive air bags and nuclear plant oxygen control, among many other uses.
  - This substance has been banned in many countries such as Australia, the UK and the EU for years.
  - In Singapore it is a $500,000 fine and fifteen years in jail for the use of azodicarbonamide.
- **Chromic acid** is an inorganic acid composed of the elements chromium, oxygen and hydrogen. Chromic acid is an intermediate in chromium plating, and is also used in ceramic glazes and colored glass. Because a solution of chromic acid in sulfuric acid is a powerful oxidizing agent, it can be used to clean laboratory glassware, particularly of otherwise insoluble organic residues.
- **Dichromate** salts contain the chromate anion. Chromates and dichromates are used in chrome plating and as pigments. These substances are toxic and labeled as carcinogens. The EU has restricted their manufacture.

Artificial Flavorings

To put it plainly, these flavors are not found in nature, they are synthesized and created in a lab. Artificial flavors are top secret, proprietary trade secrets cocktails made from the approximately thirteen hundred FDA-approved food flavorings. The FDA's definition of artificial flavoring is as follows:

> The term artificial *flavor or artificial flavoring* means any substance, the function of which is to impart flavor, which is not derived from a spice, fruit or fruit juice, vegetable or vegetable juice, edible yeast, herb, bark, bud, root, leaf or similar plant material, meat, fish, poultry, eggs, dairy products, or fermentation products thereof.

(Source:
https://www.accessdata.fda.gov/scripts/cdrh/cfdocs/cfcfr/cfrsearch.cfm
?fr=501.22)

According to the USDA:

> Aliphatic acyclic and acyclic alcohols, aldehydes, ketones, carboxylic acids and related esters, lactones, ketals, and acetals comprise more than 700 of the 1,323 chemically defined flavoring substances in the United States. Additional structural categories include aromatic, heteroaromatic, and heterocyclic substances with characteristic organoleptic properties.

(Source:
https://www.ams.usda.gov/sites/default/files/media/Flavors%20nonsynt
hetic%202%20TR.pdf)

Artificial flavorings cause many reactions or symptoms but it is hard to pinpoint as companies do not have to list what ingredients or proportions go into their specific formulation. The best we get is "artificial flavor" written on the can or box.

Symptoms or problems from artificial flavorings may be as follows:

- Allergic reactions
- Chest pain
- DNA damage
- Fatigue
- Headaches
- Depression of the nervous system
- Brain damage
- Possible Carcinogen

See Appendix C for the list of all 1,300 FDA approved food flavorings.

- 8 -

BIG PHARMA ME, DADDY

Pharmakeia is a form of the Greek root word from which we get our English words pharmacy, pharmacist and pharmaceutical. In the Bible, *pharmakeia* carried with it the idea of "sorcery". Since the 1930's, modern day sorcerers, commonly known as doctors, have utilized a book called the *Physician's Desk Reference.* This reference contains almost 300,000 drugs and, except for a few antibiotics, NONE of them cure anything—they only mask symptoms. It appears the cause of most chronic illness and allergy conditions is roughly 20% genetics and 80% environmental exposure.

In this section, we will look a few details of the pharmaceutical industry and a specific few drugs. Again, this exercise is to teach you some basic information and, more importantly, to take control of your own health and life. Do not blindly do whatever some doctor says because he has a fancy title next to his name. If your doctor does not ask you about your lifestyle, diet symptoms, past procedures and just writes your prescriptions, he is not a doctor, he is a drug dealer. They do not get paid long term or get good kickbacks if you are cured and are no longer in the system.

Now that you have a little background, we will look at the history of a few pharmaceutical companies. Earlier in the book, we examined the evidence that medical malpractice is the third leading cause of death in America. It is very possible that the protocols implemented during Covid-19 were likely the number one cause of death in the US during 2020 and 2021—even before the mRNA vaccines were pushed. For-profit hospitals changed their protocols and immediately intubated patients and put them on mechanical ventilators as a first-line defense. This should only be done as a last-ditch effort, but the hospitals received $10-39,000 per patient to do so. No wonder Pfizer and Moderna want the Covid records sealed for 75 years; this would only be a natural reaction if they were hiding something… "...the love of money is the root of all evil..." (1 Timothy 6:10)

PHARMACEUTICAL COMPANIES

Following is a list of legal issues from just a few pharmaceutical companies. The cases range from fraud to bribery to embezzlement, with lies about cancer and other diseases and more. Ask yourself if they have your best intentions in mind when they produce these chemicals, GMO's, food additives, medications, etc.

PFIZER

Pfizer is a multinational pharmaceutical corporation headquartered in New York City. Over the years, the company has faced several lawsuits, bribery allegations and scandals. Below is a comprehensive list of some notable instances:

Neurontin Off-Label Marketing Lawsuit (2004): Pfizer was accused of promoting its drug Neurontin for off-label uses, which are uses not approved by the U.S. Food and Drug Administration (FDA). The company settled the lawsuit for $430 million.

Bextra Off-Label Marketing Lawsuit (2009): Pfizer faced allegations of promoting its painkiller Bextra for off-label uses and concealing safety risks associated with the drug. The company agreed to pay $2.3 billion to settle the charges.

Illegal Marketing of Lipitor (2012): Pfizer was accused of illegally marketing its cholesterol-lowering drug Lipitor by promoting it for unapproved uses and making false claims about its benefits. The company paid $491 million to settle the charges.

Zoloft Birth Defects Lawsuits (ongoing): Numerous lawsuits have been filed against Pfizer alleging that its antidepressant drug Zoloft causes birth defects when taken during pregnancy. The litigation is ongoing, with settlements reached in some cases.

Celebrex and Bextra Safety Concerns (2005): Pfizer faced scrutiny over the safety of its painkillers Celebrex and Bextra due to an increased risk of cardiovascular events. The company voluntarily withdrew Bextra from the market and added warnings to Celebrex's label.

Chantix Suicidal Behavior Controversy (2009): Pfizer's smoking cessation drug Chantix came under scrutiny due to reports of suicidal behavior and depression in some users. The FDA required Pfizer to include a "black box" warning on Chantix's label.

Illegal Marketing of Viagra (2012): Pfizer was accused of promoting its erectile dysfunction drug Viagra for unapproved uses and making false claims about its effectiveness. The company paid $190 million to settle the charges.

Foreign Bribery Allegations (2012): Pfizer faced allegations of bribing foreign officials in several countries to gain market access and increase sales. The company reached a settlement with the U.S. Department of Justice and Securities and Exchange Commission, paying $60 million in penalties.

EpiPen Price Hike Controversy (2016): Pfizer subsidiary Mylan, which acquired the rights to EpiPen, faced backlash for significantly increasing the price of the life-saving device. The controversy led to congressional hearings and public outrage.

Opioid Litigation (ongoing): Pfizer, along with other pharmaceutical companies, has been named in numerous lawsuits related to the opioid crisis in the United States. The litigation alleges that the company downplayed the risks of opioid painkillers and contributed to the epidemic.

These are just a few notable instances involving Pfizer's companies, lawsuits, bribery allegations, and scandals. It is important to note that this list is not exhaustive, as new developments and legal actions arise over time.

JOHNSON & JOHNSON

Johnson & Johnson is a multinational corporation that operates in various sectors, including pharmaceuticals. Over the years, the company has faced several lawsuits, bribery allegations, and scandals. Here is a comprehensive list of some notable instances:

Risperdal Lawsuits:
Johnson & Johnson faced numerous lawsuits related to its antipsychotic drug, Risperdal. The company was accused of downplaying the risks of the medication and promoting off-label use, particularly among children and elderly patients. Johnson & Johnson settled many of these lawsuits, paying billions of dollars in settlements.

DePuy Hip Implant Lawsuits:
DePuy Orthopaedics, a subsidiary of Johnson & Johnson, manufactured metal-on-metal hip implants that were later found to have high failure rates and caused severe complications for patients. Lawsuits alleged that the company failed to warn about the risks associated with these implants. Johnson & Johnson settled thousands of lawsuits related to the defective hip implants, resulting in significant financial settlements.

Talcum Powder Lawsuits:
Johnson & Johnson faced numerous lawsuits claiming that its talcum powder products, such as Baby Powder and Shower-to-

Shower, caused ovarian cancer in women who used them for personal hygiene. Plaintiffs alleged that the company knew about the potential risks but failed to warn consumers adequately. The company has faced both wins and losses in these lawsuits. Some cases resulted in substantial jury verdicts against Johnson & Johnson, while others were dismissed or overturned on appeal.

Opioid Crisis Involvement:
Johnson & Johnson, along with other pharmaceutical companies, faced legal action for its alleged role in fueling the opioid crisis in the United States. The company was accused of downplaying the addictive nature of opioid painkillers it produced and engaging in deceptive marketing practices. In 2021, Johnson & Johnson reached a $230 million settlement with the state of New York to resolve opioid-related claims. The company has also faced other lawsuits and legal actions related to the opioid crisis.

Bribery Allegations in Europe:
In 2011, Johnson & Johnson faced allegations of bribery in several European countries. It was accused of paying bribes to healthcare professionals to promote its products and secure contracts. The company settled these allegations by agreeing to pay fines and implementing compliance measures. However, specific details of the settlements were not publicly disclosed.

Recall of Tylenol and Other Products:
In 1982, Johnson & Johnson faced a major crisis when seven people died after consuming cyanide-laced Tylenol capsules. The incident led to a nationwide product recall and prompted significant changes in packaging and tamper-evident seals for over-the-counter medications. Johnson & Johnson's handling of the crisis was widely praised, and the company implemented new safety measures that became industry standards.

MONSANTO

Monsanto was founded in 1901 as a chemical company in St.

Louis, Missouri. Over the years, it expanded into various sectors including agriculture, biotechnology and genetically modified organisms (GMOs). Throughout its existence, Monsanto faced numerous controversies and legal challenges related to its products and business practices. Here is a compilation of some notable instances:

Agent Orange:
During the Vietnam War, Monsanto was one of several companies that produced Agent Orange, an herbicide used by the U.S. military to defoliate forests and destroy crops. Agent Orange contained dioxin, a highly toxic chemical that has been linked to various health issues in both veterans and Vietnamese civilians, discussed earlier in the book.

PCB Contamination:
Monsanto was also involved in the production of polychlorinated biphenyls (PCBs), which were widely used as coolants and insulating fluids until their ban in the late 1970s due to environmental and health concerns. Monsanto faced lawsuits from communities and individuals affected by PCB contamination in places where the chemicals were manufactured or disposed of improperly.

Genetically Modified Organisms (GMOs):
Monsanto became known for its development and commercialization of genetically modified crops such as Roundup Ready soybeans and Bt cotton. These crops were engineered to be resistant to Monsanto's herbicide Roundup (containing glyphosate) or to produce their own insecticides. The use of GMOs raised concerns about potential environmental impacts, cross-contamination with non-GMO crops, and the control of seed supply.

Roundup and Glyphosate:
One of the most significant controversies involving Monsanto is

related to its herbicide Roundup, which contains the active ingredient glyphosate. In recent years, numerous lawsuits have been filed against Monsanto (now Bayer) by individuals who claim that exposure to Roundup caused them to develop cancer, particularly non-Hodgkin lymphoma. Some juries have ruled in favor of the plaintiffs, awarding substantial damages.

Bribery Allegations:
In 2009, Monsanto was accused of engaging in bribery activities in Indonesia. The company allegedly made illegal payments to Indonesian officials to avoid environmental impact studies and gain approval for its genetically modified cotton. The case resulted in a settlement with the U.S. Securities and Exchange Commission (SEC) in 2016, where Monsanto agreed to pay a fine without admitting or denying the allegations.

GLAXOSMITHKLINE

GlaxoSmithKline (GSK) is a multinational pharmaceutical company headquartered in London. Over the years, GSK has faced several lawsuits, bribery allegations, and scandals. Here is a comprehensive list of some notable instances:

Lawsuits
Avandia Lawsuits: GSK faced numerous lawsuits related to its diabetes drug, Avandia. The drug was linked to an increased risk of heart attacks and strokes. In 2010, GSK agreed to pay $460 million to settle thousands of lawsuits.

Paxil Birth Defects Lawsuits: GSK faced lawsuits alleging that its antidepressant drug, Paxil, caused birth defects when taken during pregnancy. In 2010, GSK settled around 800 cases for $1 billion.

Off-Label Promotion Lawsuit: In 2012, GSK paid $3 billion to settle criminal and civil charges related to the illegal promotion of several drugs for unapproved uses.

Whistleblower Lawsuit: In 2014, GSK settled a whistleblower lawsuit for $105 million. The lawsuit alleged that the company engaged in illegal marketing practices for various drugs.

Bribery Allegations
China Bribery Scandal: In 2013, Chinese authorities accused GSK of bribing doctors and hospitals to promote its products. GSK admitted to "serious breaches" of Chinese law and paid a record-breaking fine of $489 million.

Bribery in Other Countries: GSK faced bribery allegations in several other countries, including the United States, Poland, Iraq and Jordan. These allegations involved improper payments made to healthcare professionals and government officials.

Scandals
Seroxat/Paxil Controversy: GSK faced criticism for downplaying the risks associated with its antidepressant drug, Seroxat (known as Paxil in the United States). The company was accused of withholding data on the drug's safety and efficacy, particularly in children and adolescents.

Tafenoquine Controversy: GSK faced scrutiny for its anti-malarial drug, tafenoquine. Critics claimed that the drug had severe side effects and questioned GSK's clinical trial practices.

Drug Pricing Controversy: GSK, along with other pharmaceutical companies, faced criticism for high drug prices. The company was accused of exploiting its market position and making essential medications unaffordable for many patients.

MERCK & CO., INC.

Merck & Co., Inc., commonly known as Merck, is an American multinational pharmaceutical company headquartered in New Jersey. It was founded in 1891 and operates in more than 140 countries worldwide. Merck is involved in the research, development, manufacturing, and marketing of a wide range of prescription drugs, vaccines, biologic therapies and animal health products.

Lawsuits

Vioxx Lawsuits: One of the most significant legal challenges faced by Merck was related to its painkiller drug called Vioxx. In 2004, Merck voluntarily withdrew Vioxx from the market due to concerns about increased risks of heart attacks and strokes associated with long-term use. Subsequently, thousands of lawsuits were filed against Merck by patients who claimed that they suffered injuries or lost loved ones due to Vioxx. In 2007, Merck agreed to pay approximately $4.85 billion to settle most of these lawsuits.

Fosamax Lawsuits: Merck has faced numerous lawsuits related to its osteoporosis drug called Fosamax (alendronate). Patients alleged that long-term use of Fosamax caused them to suffer from osteonecrosis of the jaw (ONJ) and atypical femur fractures. Merck has settled some of these lawsuits, while others are still ongoing.

NuvaRing Lawsuits: Merck, through its subsidiary Organon, was involved in lawsuits related to the contraceptive device called NuvaRing. Users claimed that NuvaRing caused serious side effects such as blood clots, strokes, and heart attacks. Merck settled thousands of these lawsuits for a total amount exceeding $100 million.

Bribery Scandals

China Bribery Investigation: In 2013, Chinese authorities launched an investigation into allegations of bribery by several multinational pharmaceutical companies, including Merck. The investigation focused on allegations that employees of these companies bribed doctors and other healthcare professionals to prescribe their drugs. Merck cooperated with the investigation and implemented measures to strengthen its compliance practices.

Ukraine Corruption Allegations: In 2017, a Ukrainian lawmaker accused Merck of engaging in corrupt practices in Ukraine. The lawmaker alleged that Merck had paid bribes to Ukrainian officials to secure favorable treatment for its products. Merck denied the allegations and stated that it adheres to strict ethical standards in all its business operations.

BAYER AG

Bayer AG is a multinational pharmaceutical and life sciences company headquartered in Germany. Over the years, Bayer has faced several lawsuits, bribery allegations, and scandals. Here is a comprehensive list of some notable instances:

Lawsuits

Roundup Lawsuits: Bayer acquired Monsanto in 2018, inheriting thousands of lawsuits related to the herbicide Roundup. The lawsuits claim that Roundup's active ingredient, glyphosate, causes cancer. As of July 2021, Bayer has settled or resolved around 125,000 claims for approximately $11 billion.

Yaz/Yasmin Lawsuits: Bayer faced numerous lawsuits related to its birth control pills Yaz and Yasmin. The lawsuits alleged that the pills caused blood clots, leading to serious health complications. Bayer settled thousands of cases for over $2 billion.

Trasylol Lawsuits: Trasylol was a drug used to control bleeding during heart surgeries. Bayer faced thousands of lawsuits claiming that Trasylol caused kidney damage and increased the risk of death. In 2010, Bayer agreed to pay $60 million to settle most of the cases.

Baycol Lawsuits: Baycol was a cholesterol-lowering drug that was withdrawn from the market in 2001 due to reports of severe muscle toxicity and deaths. Bayer faced numerous lawsuits from patients who suffered adverse effects. The company settled thousands of cases for over $1 billion.

Bribery Allegations

Latin America Bribery Allegations: In 2009, Bayer faced allegations of bribery in Latin America. It was reported that the company paid bribes to government officials and doctors to promote its products. The U.S. Securities and Exchange Commission (SEC) investigated the matter, and in 2016, Bayer agreed to pay $5.6 million to settle the charges.

China Bribery Allegations: In 2013, Chinese authorities launched an investigation into allegations that Bayer employees bribed doctors to prescribe its drugs. The investigation resulted in several arrests and fines for the company. Bayer cooperated with the authorities and implemented stricter compliance measures.

South Korea Bribery Allegations: In 2017, Bayer faced allegations of bribery in South Korea. It was reported that the company made improper payments to doctors to boost sales of its drugs. The Korean Fair Trade Commission fined Bayer approximately $2.6 million for violating anti-trust laws.

Scandals

Contaminated Blood Scandal: In the 1980s, Bayer's subsidiary, Cutter Biological, sold blood-clotting products contaminated with HIV and hepatitis C. Thousands of hemophiliacs who used these products were infected, leading to numerous deaths. Bayer faced multiple lawsuits and paid millions of dollars in settlements.

Contraceptive Pill Scandal: In the 1990s, Bayer faced a scandal related to its contraceptive pills. It was revealed that the company had knowingly sold millions of defective birth control pills in Europe, resulting in unintended pregnancies and health risks for women. Bayer faced legal action and paid compensation to affected individuals.

Price-Fixing Scandal: In 2001, Bayer was involved in a price-fixing scandal related to vitamins. The company conspired with other pharmaceutical companies to artificially inflate prices, leading to higher costs for consumers and healthcare providers. Bayer pleaded guilty and paid a $66 million fine.

BRISTOL-MYERS SQUIBB

Bristol-Myers Squibb (BMS) is a global biopharmaceutical company that specializes in the research, development, and manufacturing of prescription drugs. Over the years, the company has faced several legal issues, including lawsuits, bribery allegations, and scandals. Here is a comprehensive list of some notable instances:

Securities Fraud Lawsuit (2002)
In 2002, BMS faced a securities fraud lawsuit filed by shareholders. The lawsuit alleged that the company engaged in fraudulent accounting practices to inflate its revenue and stock price. BMS settled the case for $300 million without admitting any wrongdoing.

Plavix Patent Litigation (2006-2012)
BMS was involved in a series of patent litigations related to its

blockbuster drug Plavix. The company faced challenges from generic manufacturers who claimed that BMS's patents were invalid or unenforceable. These litigations resulted in settlements and licensing agreements with various generic companies.

Illegal Marketing Practices (2007)
BMS faced allegations of illegal marketing practices related to its antipsychotic drug Abilify. The company was accused of promoting off-label uses of the drug and providing kickbacks to healthcare professionals for prescribing it. BMS settled the case for $515 million.

Foreign Corrupt Practices Act Violation (2010)
In 2010, BMS settled charges with the U.S. Securities and Exchange Commission (SEC) for violating the Foreign Corrupt Practices Act (FCPA). The company was accused of making improper payments to healthcare professionals in various countries to increase sales of its products. BMS paid a $14 million penalty to settle the charges.

Plavix False Claims Act Lawsuit (2011)
BMS faced a False Claims Act lawsuit alleging that it promoted Plavix for off-label uses and made false statements about its safety and efficacy. The lawsuit also claimed that BMS paid kickbacks to healthcare providers. The case was settled for $75 million.

Hepatitis C Drug Pricing Controversy (2015)
BMS faced criticism for the high pricing of its hepatitis C drug, Sovaldi. The drug was priced at $1,000 per pill, leading to concerns about accessibility and affordability. The controversy sparked a broader debate on the pricing of life-saving medications.

Opdivo Clinical Trial Misconduct (2018)
BMS faced allegations of clinical trial misconduct related to its cancer drug Opdivo. It was reported that the company failed to disclose safety data from a clinical trial, potentially putting patients

at risk. BMS acknowledged the oversight and took corrective actions.

Opioid Marketing Investigation (Ongoing)

BMS is currently under investigation by several U.S. states regarding its marketing practices for opioid painkillers. The investigation aims to determine if the company downplayed the risks of addiction and overstated the benefits of its opioid products.

ABBOTT LABORATORIES

Abbott Laboratories is a multinational healthcare company that specializes in the development, manufacturing, and marketing of pharmaceuticals, medical devices, diagnostics and nutrition products.

Lawsuits

Off-Label Marketing Lawsuit: In 2012, Abbott Laboratories agreed to pay $1.5 billion to settle allegations of off-label marketing of its drug Depakote. The company was accused of promoting the drug for uses not approved by the U.S. Food and Drug Administration (FDA), including the treatment of dementia and schizophrenia.

False Claims Act Settlement: Abbott Laboratories reached a $700 million settlement with the U.S. government in 2012 over allegations of illegal marketing practices related to its drugs Depakote, TriCor and Niaspan. The company was accused of promoting these drugs for off-label uses and paying kickbacks to healthcare professionals.

Securities Fraud Lawsuit: Abbott Laboratories faced a securities fraud lawsuit in 2008 related to allegations that it misled investors about the safety risks associated with its diet drug Meridia. The company agreed to pay $22.5 million to settle the lawsuit.

Qui Tam Lawsuit: Abbott Laboratories settled a qui tam lawsuit in 2003 for $622 million. The lawsuit alleged that the company engaged in illegal pricing practices by inflating drug prices and defrauding Medicaid programs.

Bribery Scandals

Bribery Allegations in Russia: In 2011, Abbott Laboratories faced allegations of bribery in Russia. It was reported that the company paid bribes to government officials to secure contracts and gain market access. The U.S. Securities and Exchange Commission (SEC) investigated the matter, but no charges were filed against the company.

Bribery Allegations in China: Abbott Laboratories was also implicated in a bribery scandal in China in 2013. The company was accused of bribing doctors and hospital administrators to increase sales of its products. Abbott cooperated with the Chinese authorities during the investigation, and several employees were disciplined or terminated as a result.

Scandals

Infant Formula Scandal: Abbott Laboratories faced a scandal in 2010 related to its infant formula products in China. The company was accused of selling contaminated formula that led to the death of several infants. Abbott recalled the affected products and implemented stricter quality control measures.

Misleading Advertising Scandal: In 2009, Abbott Laboratories faced criticism for misleading advertising related to its weight loss product, Ensure. The company was accused of making false claims about the effectiveness of the product in helping consumers lose weight. Abbott agreed to modify its advertising practices following an investigation by the Federal Trade Commission (FTC).

Drug Pricing Scandal: Abbott Laboratories was involved in a drug pricing scandal in 2001. The company was accused of inflating drug prices and overcharging government healthcare programs, resulting in higher costs for consumers and taxpayers. Abbott settled the allegations by paying $100 million to various states and federal agencies.

ABBVIE INC.

AbbVie Inc. is a global biopharmaceutical company that focuses on the discovery, development and commercialization of innovative therapies in various therapeutic areas, including immunology, oncology, neuroscience, and virology.

Lawsuits

Humira Patent Litigation: AbbVie has faced several lawsuits related to its blockbuster drug Humira, which is used to treat autoimmune diseases such as rheumatoid arthritis and Crohn's disease. The company has been accused of engaging in anti-competitive practices to maintain its monopoly on the drug by filing numerous patents and entering into settlement agreements with generic manufacturers.

AndroGel Marketing Practices: In 2014, AbbVie was sued by the Federal Trade Commission (FTC) for allegedly engaging in anti-competitive practices to delay the entry of generic versions of its testosterone replacement therapy drug, AndroGel. The company was accused of filing baseless patent infringement lawsuits against potential generic competitors.

Depakote Off-Label Marketing: Abbott Laboratories, which later spun off AbbVie as a separate entity, faced legal action related to the off-label marketing of its epilepsy drug Depakote. The company was accused of promoting the drug for uses not approved by the U.S. Food and Drug Administration (FDA), including the treatment of dementia and schizophrenia.

Bribery Scandals

Foreign Corrupt Practices Act (FCPA) Investigation: In 2018, AbbVie disclosed that it was under investigation by the U.S. Department of Justice (DOJ) and Securities and Exchange Commission (SEC) for potential violations of the FCPA. The investigation focused on the company's interactions with foreign government officials and healthcare professionals in various countries.

China Bribery Allegations: In 2013, Chinese authorities announced an investigation into allegations of bribery by several multinational pharmaceutical companies, including Abbott Laboratories (AbbVie's former parent company). The investigation alleged that the company had bribed doctors and other healthcare professionals to prescribe its drugs.

Conclusion

Even a cursory review of the information in this chapter shows that there are a lot of really scary practices going on in an industry that is not taking patient health into consideration by purposely using deceptive practices, purposely putting out products that cause more harm than good and willingly and consistently participating in scandalous behavior and bribery, often in countries that are known to have very poor human rights standards. Great consideration and research should go into any of these drugs and the company that produces them before a medication is taken.

(Source:
https://en.wikipedia.org/wiki/List_of_largest_pharmaceutical_settlements)

- 9 -

STATIN DRUGS & CHRONIC ILLNESS

Our next big offender comes from one of Merck's most prolific patents, lovastatin. The history of statins begins in 1976 when a Japanese biochemist isolated a factor from the fungus *Penicillium citrinum* which he identified as an inhibitor of HMG-CoA reductase. This substance, which he named "compactin" or "mevastatin", was the first statin to be administered to humans.

(Source: Hajar R. Statins: past and present. Heart Views. 2011 Jul;12(3):121-7. doi: 10.4103/1995-705X.95070. PMID: 22567201; PMCID: PMC3345145)

Merck began clinical trials of lovastatin in April 1980, in correlation with a dramatic uptick in propaganda regarding cholesterol. "Cholesterol" started becoming a buzzword at this time and coincidentally, dietary guidelines started appearing in the early 1980's TV commercials, news, magazines and other media claiming cholesterol causes heart attacks and strokes. Fear campaigns always work, and tyrants never stop using them because they are so effective.

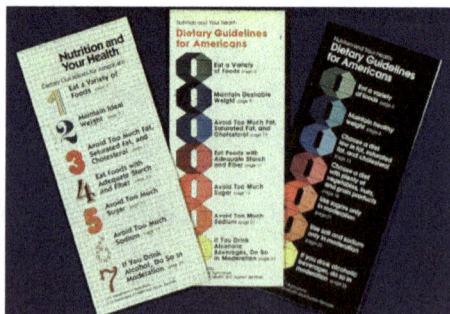

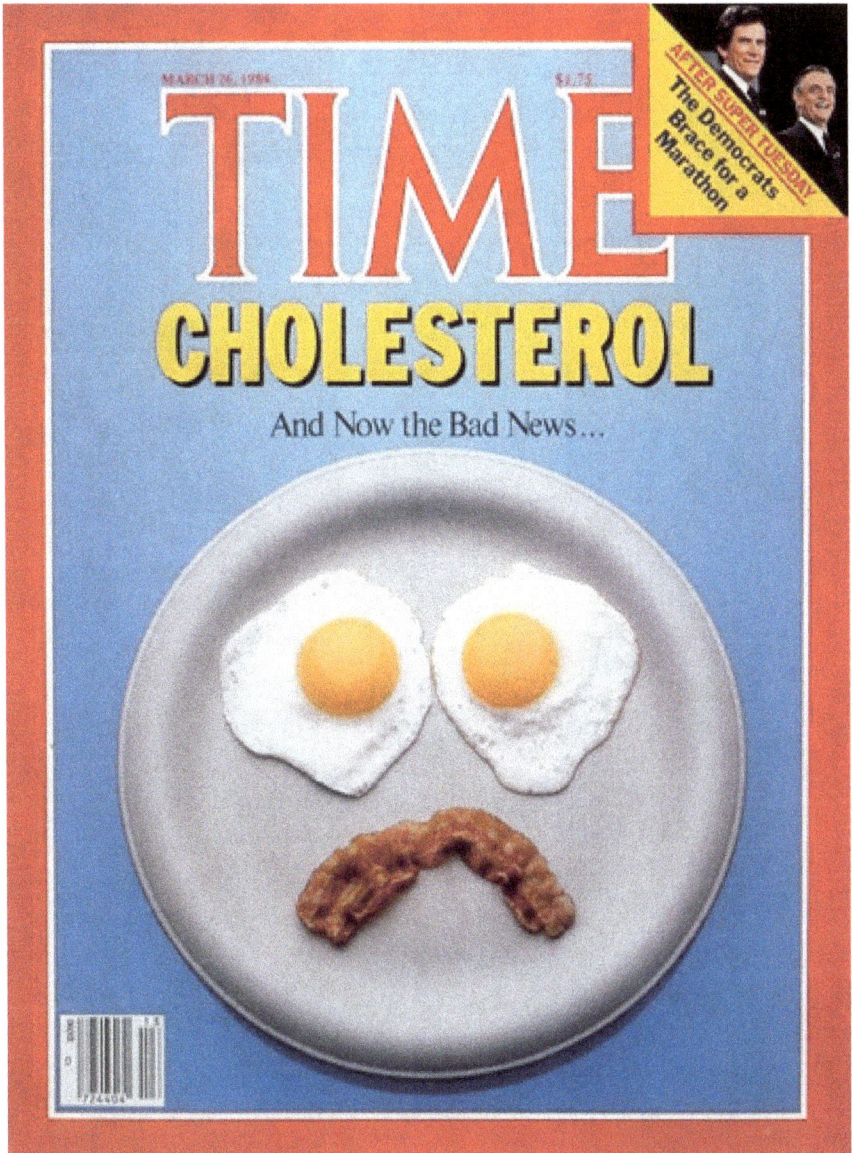

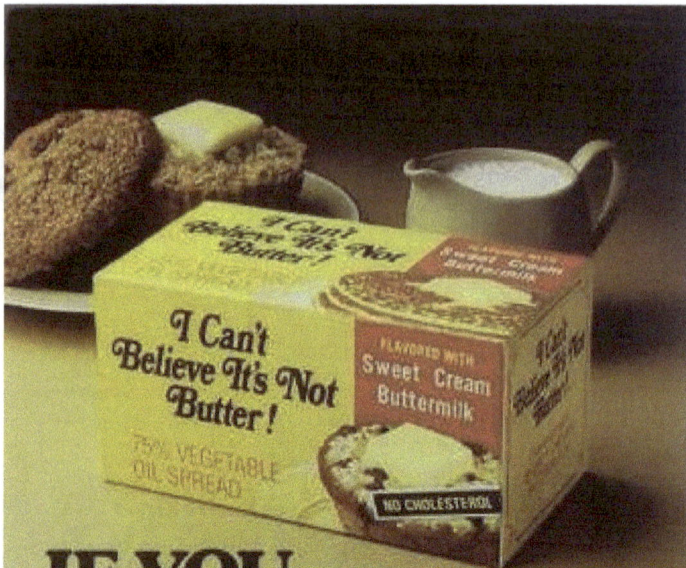

IF YOU LOVE BUTTER BUT HATE CHOLESTEROL!

- You'll love "I Can't Believe It's Not Butter!".
- It tastes like butter because it's flavored with sweet cream buttermilk!
- But unlike butter and butter blends, *it contains no cholesterol!*

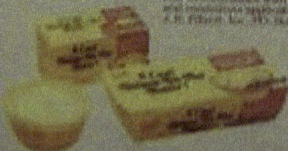

SAVE 15¢ on 1 lb. (stick or soft) of "I Can't Believe It's Not Butter!".

40600 102152

After so many years of the media, government and big corporations pushing a fear campaign and waging an information war on cholesterol during the trial phase of lovastatin (1980-1987), suddenly a solution appeared.

On September 1, 1987, lovastatin became the first statin to be approved in the United States by the FDA. This agent is responsible for revolutionizing the treatment of hypercholesterolemia, eventually achieving peak annual sales of more than $1 billion. It is almost as if all the media, big corporations and government knew about the statin trials and were seeking to profit off of the drug approval...

Simvastatin, a side-chain ester analog of lovastatin, was approved for marketing in Sweden in 1988, with subsequent worldwide distribution. The approval and distribution of this drug was followed by pravastatin in 1991, fluvastatin in 1994, atorvastatin in 1997, cerivastatin in 1998, and rosuvastatin in 2003, all also under various brand name labels.

Research shows that cholesterol is not "the cause" of heart attacks and strokes but when your doctors scare you into taking these drugs for these claims, you tend to take them. Too many people have been scared into thinking their doctor with his credentials is the pinnacle of medical knowledge and that his opinion is their only option.

Statins pose a very serious risk because they strip the body of essential cholesterol. The brain is comprised of 25% cholesterol and the nerve sheaths, called myelin, are also comprised of cholesterol. Myelin is basically insulation for your nerves and statin drugs cause demyelination. When it is worn away or damaged, nerves can deteriorate, causing problems in the brain and throughout the body.

Alzheimer's Disease and dementia may be pharmaceutically-induced diseases directly from statin drug use, which would also correlate to the timeline of the dramatic jump of Alzheimer's Disease and dementia increases in the past few decades. My own father developed PolyMyalgia Rheumatica (PMR), also called statin-induced myalgia and myositis, rhabdomyolysis, myalgia or mild hyperCKemia.

Additionally, cholesterol is a steroid hormone that is responsible for all the sex hormones: testosterone, estrogen, progesterone etc. If cholesterol is not available to help synthesize the hormones, there will be significant other issues cropping up in growth and development, reproduction and aging.

For further reading, review this study on Pubmed.gov: "Self-limited toxic statin myopathy, Immune-mediated necrotizing myopathy and anti-HMGCR antibodies".

(Source: ncbi.nlm.nih.gov/pmc/articles/PMC6019601/)

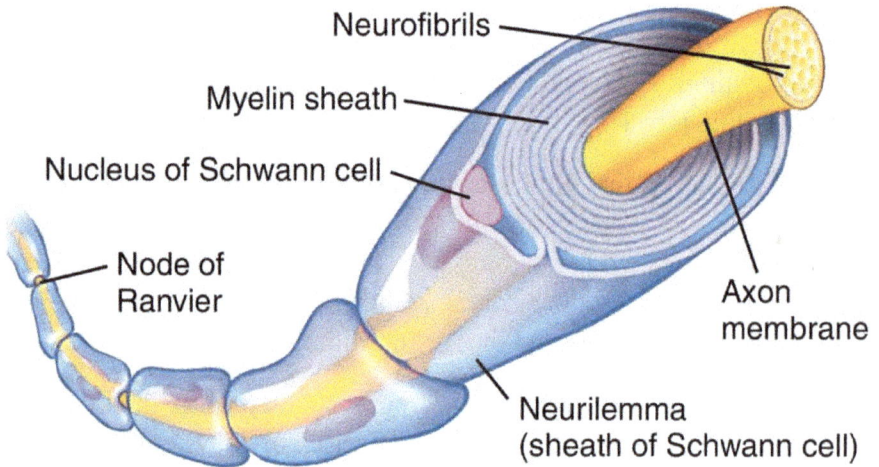

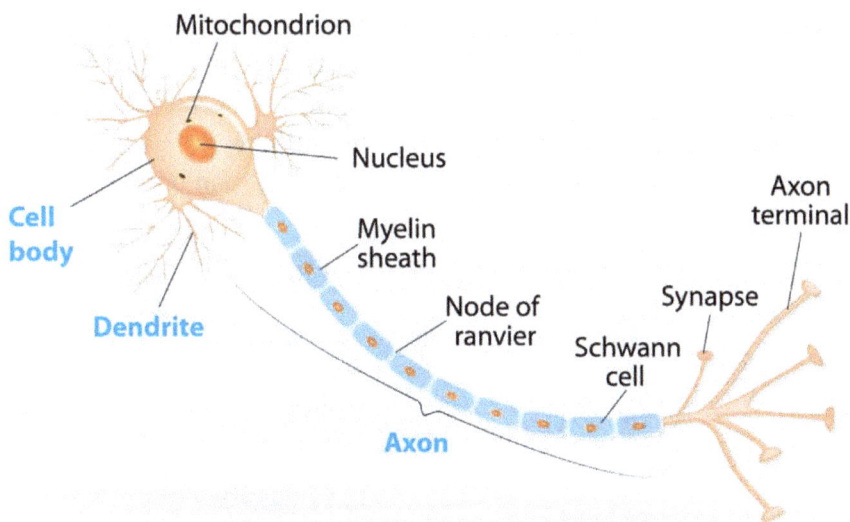

The Statin Connection: Alzheimer's & Dementia

The majority of these wide-spread pharmaceuticals pose a huge risk, as seen in the bulky side effects inserts that come with any medication you take or when the TV commercials list all the side effects and complications that come from these drugs. Many of these illnesses can be cured with simple nutrition modifications, lifestyle changes and by eliminating environmental toxins instead of these drugs that cause irreparable damage or death. Doctors are not taught nutritional cures, natural remedies, integrative medicine or homeopathic medicine to get to the root cause of your illness. The doctor's primary job is to prescribe a drug to mask the symptoms and keep you in the system.

It is very hard to find any Alzheimer's and dementia statistics at all and those that are available only go back to 1995 for Alzheimer's and 2010 for dementia. This would indicate that this trend is a relatively new phenomenon that began around the late 1980's—the same time statin drugs were approved.

Again, it appears the powers-that-be are suppressing information on these major topics, as Alzheimer's and dementia care is big business. These companies profit so much from you or your loved one being sick and in the medical system. Going by the track record of pharmaceutical companies, the patterns are not hard to find. Destroying the lives of everyday people is acceptable collateral damage to companies bringing in billions of dollars and manipulating the government for their own use and protection.

Alzheimer's Cost and Funding 2010 -2050

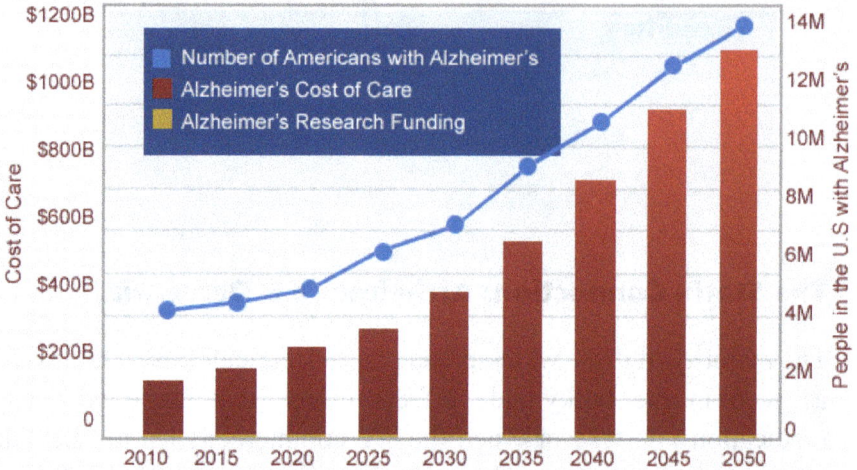

Source: Alzheimer's Study Group. A National Alzheimer's Strategic Plan: The Report of the Alzheimer's Studt Group (March 2009); Alzheimer's Association, Changing the Trajectory of Alzheimer's Disease: A National Imperative (May 2010); National Institute of Health Office of the Budget website.

A bulging burden

Estimated number of people with dementia* worldwide
2010 — 36m
2030 — 66m
2050 — 115m

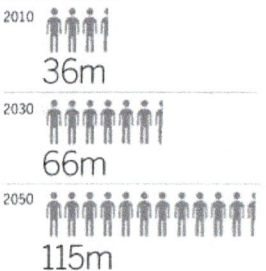

Estimated social, medical and care costs per person with dementia* (2010)
$17,000

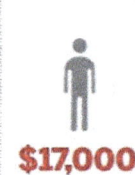

Estimated global costs of dementia* (2010, $bn)
Informal care: 252
Social costs: 256
Medical costs: 96
Total = **$604bn**

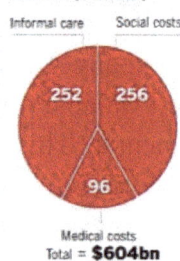

Total size of seven biggest Alzheimer's drugs markets**
2011 — $5.8bn
2020 — $14.5bn

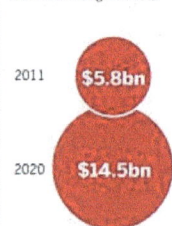

* Alzheimer's is the most common cause of dementia ** US, Japan, France, Germany, Italy, Spain, UK   Sources: Alzheimer's Disease International; Datamonitor   FT graphic

THE COST OF DEMENTIA IN THE UK

- PRIVATELY FUNDED SOCIAL CARE
- CARE PROVIDED DIRECTLY BY FAMILIES
- PUBLICLY FUNDED SOCIAL CARE (NHS)
- DIAGNOSES, OTHER & HEALTHCARE COSTS

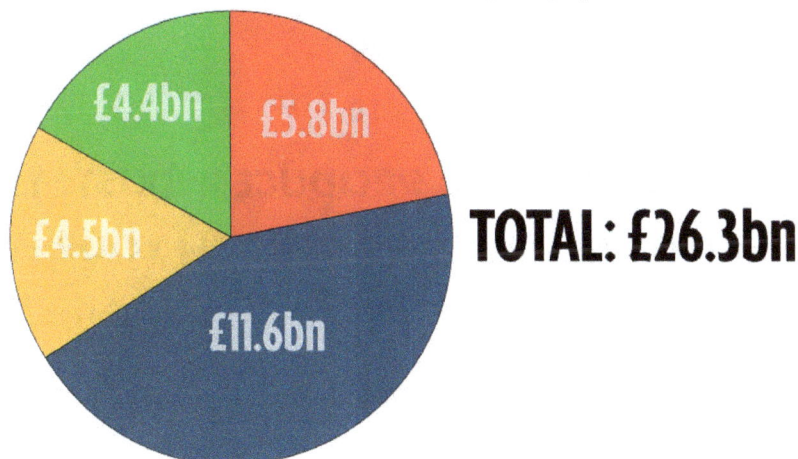

£4.4bn
£5.8bn
£4.5bn
£11.6bn

TOTAL: £26.3bn

SOURCE: ALZHEIMER'S SOCIETY

Alzheimer's Disease Projections
Cost of Care (in Billions)

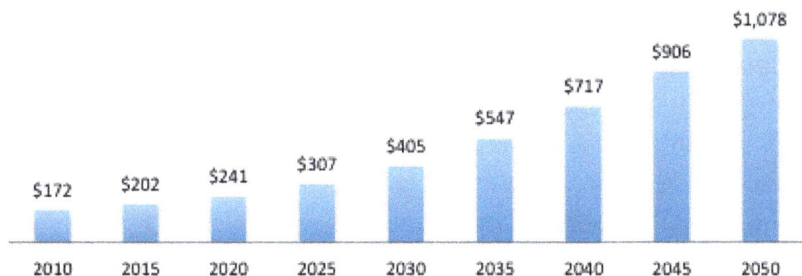

$172 (2010), $202 (2015), $241 (2020), $307 (2025), $405 (2030), $547 (2035), $717 (2040), $906 (2045), $1,078 (2050)

www.Senior-Care-Resources.com

MEAT, DAIRY & PRODUCE INDUSTRY:
EAT YOUR VACCINES & FINISH YOUR LAB GROWN MEAT

Keep in mind that all of our food has been tampered with—from the fertilizers to the seeds, to the produce itself and at every step of the meat and dairy industries. There is almost nothing untouched.

PRODUCE: Grow and Eat Your Vaccines!

Farmland in the US is not under the care and management it is assumed to be. Bill Gates, yes, the computer nerd, owns more US farmland than any other private entity in our country. Foreign nationals and foreign countries are allowed to monopolize our land and industry. In Arizona for instance, Saudi Arabia owns huge parcels and grows alfalfa crops--a water-heavy crop. They are given priority by the local government to grow this crop. Saudia Arabia does this in America because they have banned growing alfalfa in their own country. The crops are grown in the US, to the detriment of American citizens, and then the crop is shipped to Saudi Arabia for cattle feed—at the convenience of Saudia Arabia.

Bill Gates, the same guy who said we need to depopulate the world, has been buying up farmland at an alarming rate. The formula from his 2010 "Innovating to Zero" conference was:

$$CO_2 = P \times S \times E \times C$$

- P = People
- S = Service per person
- E = Energy per person
- C = CO_2 per energy unit

Gates stated one or more factors need to be zero. Keep in mind that WE are the "carbon" the elites want to eliminate. Also keep in mind that Bill Gates has no university level degrees or credentials, much less medical or science credentials—the man does not even have a bachelor's degree in computer science.

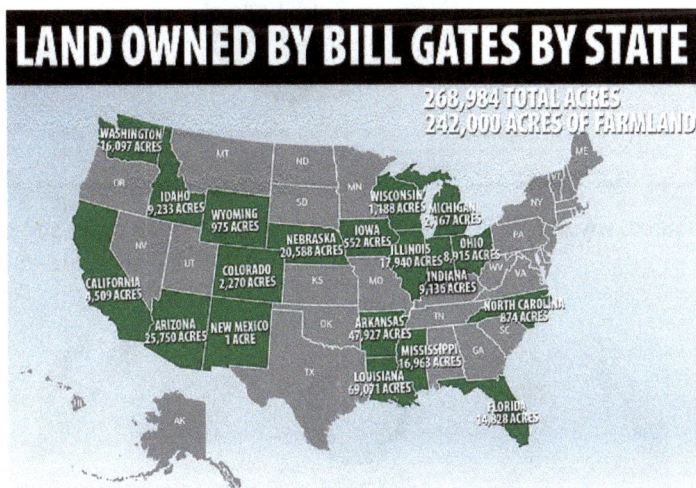

(Source: www.eastcoastdaily.in/2021/01/19/bill-gates-titled-also-as-americas-biggest-farmland-owner.html)

During this same speech in 2010, Gates said **"The world today has 6.8 billion people. That's headed up to about 9 billion. Now if we do a really great job on new vaccines, healthcare, reproductive health services, we could lower that by, perhaps, 10 or 15%."**

(Source: https://www.reuters.com/article/factcheck-gates-vaccine-idUSL1N2MF1L8)

This is the same Bill Gates who has pushed vaccines and done horrific vaccine studies in Africa. He has recently funded a company that produced "Apeel", a produce sealant that contains undisclosed ingredients that are to "protect" foods such as organic avocado, apples, oranges and cucumbers from premature spoilage.

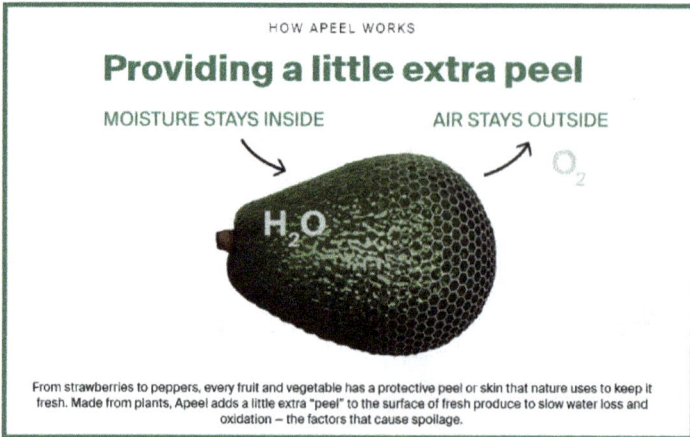

(Source: www.foodengineeringmag.com/articles/98080-apeel-and-natures-pride-team-up-to-extend-avocado-shelf-life-in-europe)

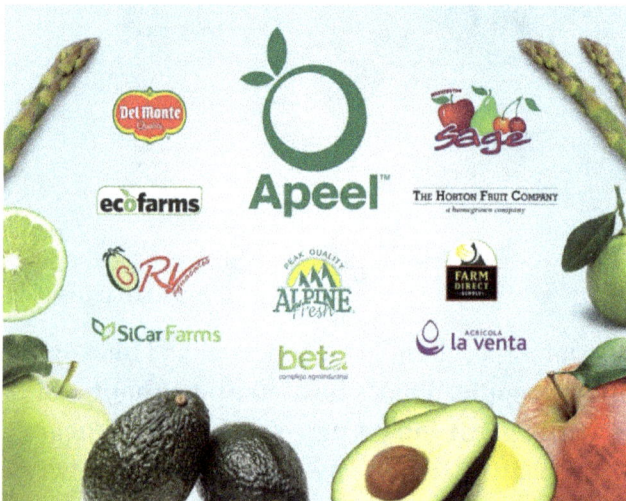

(Source: www.fruitnet.com/eurofruit/apeel-unveils-supplier-network/179496.article)

This very well could be introduced in anticipation of mRNA vaccines being inserted into these food items as a way to preserve the vaccines inside them, not the produce. That is why it is being used on food items you eat raw, so the mRNA vaccine is not harmed by cooking. If you say that is far-fetched, University of California, Riverside has produced lettuce that contains mRNA vaccines, so get ready, you are going to take the mRNA vaccine whether you like it or not. They have already been using it in pigs and are rolling it out in poultry and cattle next, if it is not already in place.

(Source: www.universityofcalifornia.edu/news/grow-and-eat-your-own-vaccines)

Here are a few quotes from some articles on mRNA produce:

> The future of vaccines may look more like eating a salad than getting a shot in the arm." UC Riverside scientists are studying whether they can turn edible plants like lettuce into mRNA vaccine factories.

(Source: universityofcalifornia.edu/news/grow-and-eat-your-own-vaccines)

Here is another quote from another researcher from an article titled "Lettuce, the new secret weapon for making vaccines cheaper in the developing world".

> If we take insulin directly orally, we have enzymes in the stomach which will degrade the protein," explained Daniell. "Insulin is a hormone, which is a protein, and it will never reach the blood stream. Any plant cell has a cell wall that protects this protein from digestion, it will be safely taken to the gut, where it will be absorbed.

(Source: www.universityofcalifornia.edu/news/grow-and-eat-your-own-vaccines)

Daniell's lab also produces vaccines against infectious diseases, for example polio, tuberculosis, and malaria, and their production method is very different from what's currently available.

> "Take polio. There has been a polio outbreak in Southeast Asia. It has jumped to Africa.

Unfortunately, it was vaccine derived," said Daniell. He added that the outbreak was blamed on vaccine storage, because correct refrigeration was not provided, and the virus in the vaccine mutated. "Having a whole virus or bacteria in the vaccine is not good. We don't use a whole virus or bacteria," he explained.

(Source: whyy.org/segments/lettuce-the-new-secret-weapon-for-making-vaccines-cheaper-in-the-developing-world/)

There are already companies growing, and manufacturing this Produce of Death, and with the history of our government I would assume they have been testing this out on us for years, so take care with foods you eat raw.

As a side note, the true motive behind the globalists' depopulation agenda is not because of climate change, social justice or any other nonsense. The world governments want to consolidate power under one world ruler (Satan, via the Antichrist) but the population has become too numerous and too aware of their treachery so they must make the population too sick, ignorant and reduced to fight back effectively. They will continue to manufacture crises to take our freedoms and we will trade them for a minor convenience.

MEAT & DAIRY INDUSTRY

The meat and dairy industries are another giant monopoly with just a handful of companies that own all of the major livestock, meat processing and dairy operations in this country and a great deal of them are not even owned by *American* companies. A foreign company owning half of our major stockyards is clearly a national security risk, yet our government takes no action to look into this, much less prevent it.

The top four meat processing companies in the US are seen in the graphic below. These big four processors are:

1. Cargill, a global commodity trader based in Minnesota;
2. Tyson Foods Inc., the chicken producer that is the biggest US meat company by sales;
3. JBS SA, the world's biggest meatpacker, based in Brazil;
4. National Beef Packing Co., which is controlled by Brazilian beef producer Marfrig Global Foods

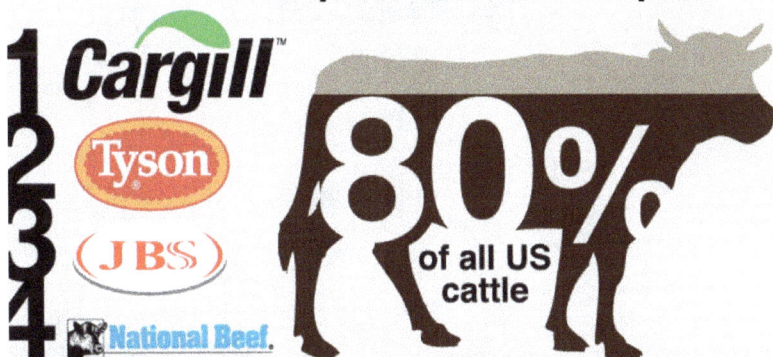

Top 4 US Beef Companies

From Foodopoly: The Battle Over the Future of Food and Farming in America by Wenonah Hauter / foodopoly.org

(Source: www.europe.chinadaily.com.cn/photo/2014-
07/14/content_17762807_2.htm)

There are many hidden dangers in the meat and dairy industry that
are hard to get around. The industry uses a lot of vaccines—around
29 million pounds in 2011 alone—and these contain heavy metals,
live viruses and now mRNA technology that has not been
thoroughly studied.

In addition to this, meat animals are also given growth hormones,
hormones to lay eggs and hormones to keep producing milk. The
food the cattle are being fed contains GMO's, pesticides and
herbicides at much larger rates than what is acceptable for human
consumption. These animals are also pumped full of anabolic
steroids, insulin-like growth hormone (IFG-1), beta-adrenergic
receptor agonists/antagonists—all things that are meant to raise
profits and decrease regulatory "climate control" metrics and have
nothing to do with actually improving your health.

The optimal route to procure meat animals is to raise your own, but as this is not practical for the vast majority, buying from local farmers is one of the best options. Make sure the meat is certified organic, non-GMO, grassfed and finished. Do not be deceived by fake marketing ploys that say things like "natural", "simple ingredients", "sustainable", "keto", "paleo", "no added hormones" and/or "grass-fed" as they mean nothing and, in many cases, dupe people into paying more for the exact same product.

Below is a photo of a commercial poultry farm. The birds have been given so many hormones that their breasts grow so large that the bird cannot move and is crippled and deformed. There are anecdotal stories of the bird's legs breaking from the sheer weight of their disproportional weights.

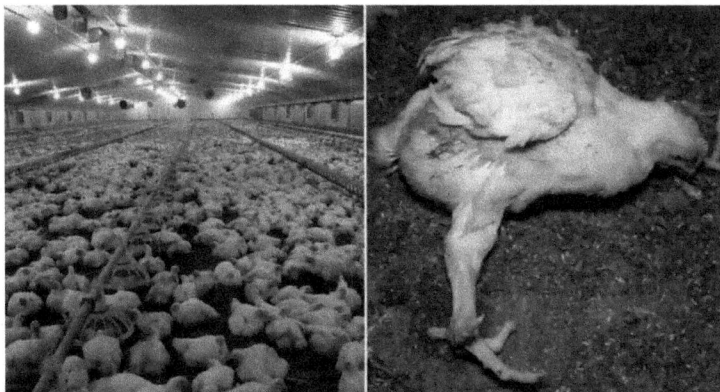

Other concerns in this industry are the presence of antibiotic resistant strains of bacteria such as E. coli, salmonella and campylobacter. Many vaccines contain mercury, aluminum and formaldehyde. From our friends at Monsanto comes recombinant bovine growth hormone (rBGH), a synthetic hormone that is marketed to dairy farmers to increase milk production in cows. It has been used in the US since it was approved by the FDA in 1993, but its use is not permitted in the EU, Canada and some other countries.

Below is what we currently know about rBGH:

- rBGH has been declared unsafe by medical experts

- o Many milk producers have stopped using this due to safety concerns, but it has not been widely banned
- rBGH is a danger to humans
    - o As it also contains insulin like growth factor (IGF-1), there are studies showing links to greater risk of breast, prostate, colorectal and even lung cancers
- Potential link to diabetes
    - o Monsanto, with support from the FDA stated rBGH would not transfer through milk but medical cases have shown otherwise with one case in particular showing the link between rBGH and diabetes onset in an otherwise healthy bodybuilder
- Potential milk contamination, mastitis and need for antibiotics
    - o Milk with rBGH is more likely to become contaminated and has since been banned in the EU and elsewhere
    - o rBGH can cause mastitis and inflammation in the cows, increasing bacterial and even pus contaminants in the milk

(Source: explore.globalhealing.com/8-shocking-facts-bovine-growth-hormone)

Most producers label their milk with rBGH and rBST so finding milk without these additions is advisable. Optimally, buying organic or raw milk and goat's milk are your best options.

LAB GROWN MEAT

Another concerning trend is globalist leaders who are trying to shut down world farming and meat consumption as they say it is causing global warming and, now, climate change. As a result, they are imposing unrealistic environmental goals and shutting down farms. This is happening in America as well, but it is not making the news yet. New regulations being imposed will cause small meat packers to have to conform to new nitrogen emission laws that will effectively put them out of business unless they upgrade with millions of dollars' worth of equipment and testing protocols.

As if all these things were not concerning enough, enter the era of lab-grown meat. New companies are coming online that are "growing" meat cells in giant bioreactors and selling to consumers.

> The US company Good Meat said the bioreactors would grow more than 13,000 tons of chicken and beef a year. It will use cells taken from cell banks or eggs, so the meat will not require the slaughter of any livestock.
>
> There are about 170 companies around the world working on cultured meat, but Good Meat is the only company to have gained regulatory approval to sell its product to the public. It began serving cultivated chicken in Singapore in December 2020.
>
> (Source: www.theguardian.com/environment/2022/may/25/worlds-largest-vats-for-growing-no-kill-meat-to-be-built-in-us)

Many companies are 3D printing this "meat product" and in the US, many companies are gearing up for mass production.

> Israeli-based company Believer Meats is commencing its first U.S. commercial facility in North Carolina. Located in Wilson, the company's new spurt will be the biggest and largest cultivated production facility established so far, covering a site of 200,000-square-[feet...]
>
> Believer Meats is one of the largest companies producing lab-grown meat with non-GMO animal cells. The company is cruelty-free and very respectful of the ecological environment. With the 10,000 metric tons of cultivated meat capacity, Believer Meats seems to be about to change the industry.
>
> "Our facility propels Believer forward as a leader in the cultivated meat industry," says Nicole Johnson-Hoffman, CEO of Believer Meats, in the press release.
>
> (Source: www.interestingengineering.com/innovation/worlds-largest-3d-printed-meat-facility

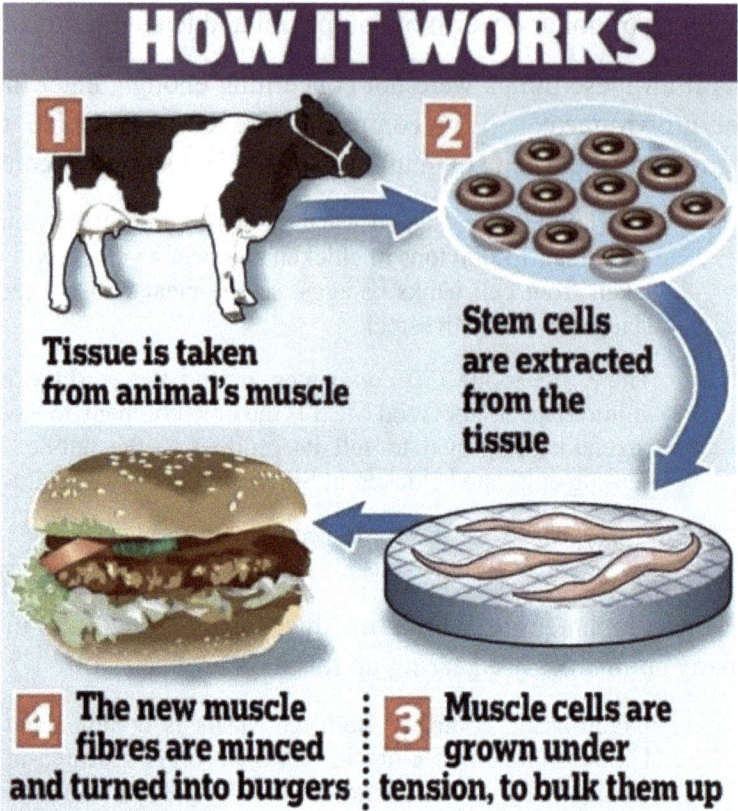

HOW IT WORKS

1 Tissue is taken from animal's muscle

2 Stem cells are extracted from the tissue

3 Muscle cells are grown under tension, to bulk them up

4 The new muscle fibres are minced and turned into burgers

(Source: www.steemit.com/food/@victor-lucas/the-potential-of-lab-grown-meat)

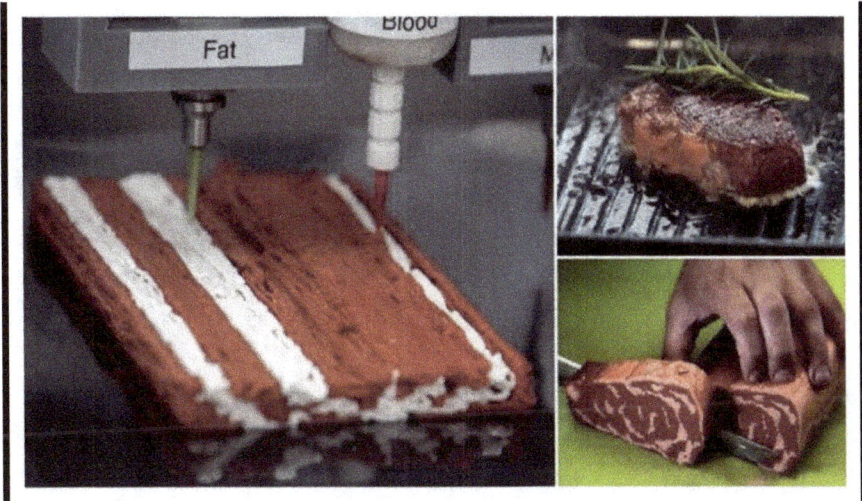

(Source: www.metro.co.uk/2020/06/30/worlds-first-3d-printed-vegan-steak-hitting-restaurants-soon-12924017/)

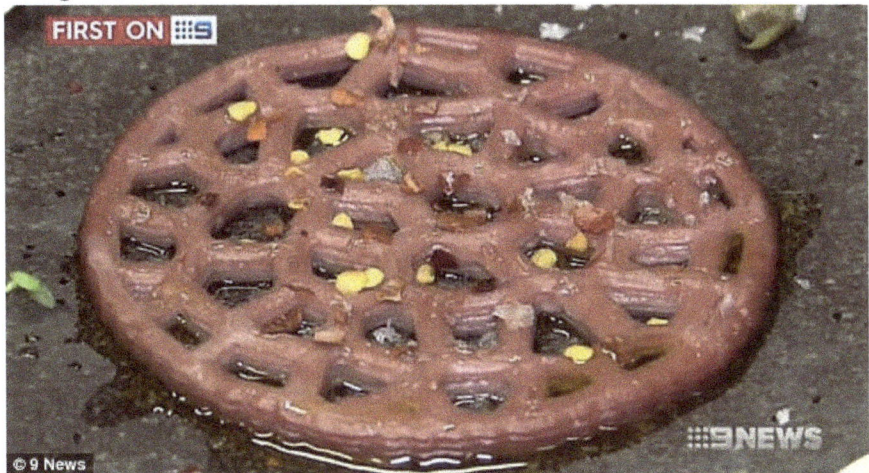

This is an image of lab grown meat, it can be 3D printed into any shape.

(Source: www.dailymail.co.uk/news/article-4468296/New-3D-printed-meat-exhibited-Melbourne.html)

(Source for following page: www.dailymail.co.uk/sciencetech/article-6826961/UK-scientists-join-race-lab-grown-meat-Pig-cells-cultured-blades-grass.html)

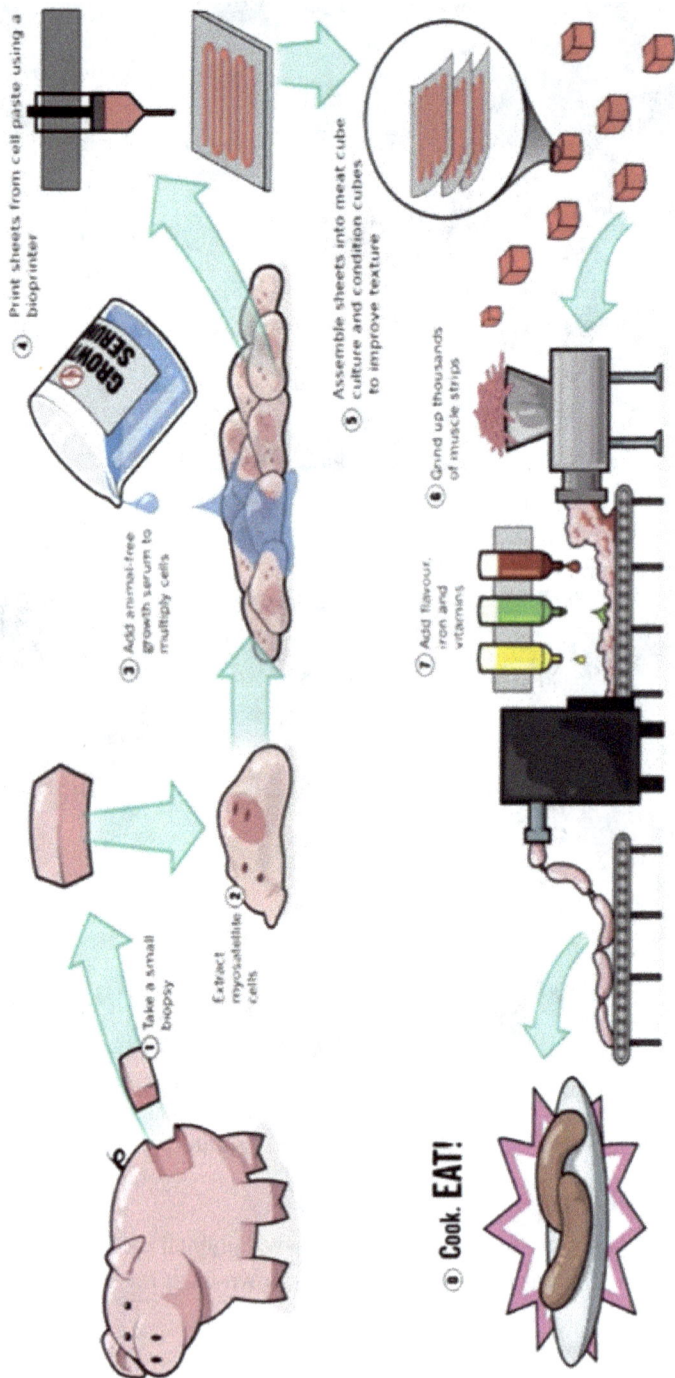

① Take a small biopsy

② Add animal-free growth serum to multiply cells

③ Extract myosatellite cells

④ Print sheets from cell paste using a bioprinter

⑤ Assemble sheets into meat cube culture and condition cubes to improve texture

⑥ Grind up thousands of muscle strips

⑦ Add flavour, iron and vitamins

⑧ Cook. EAT!

GROWTH SERUM

- 11 -

THIRSTY? HAVE A NICE COLD GLASS OF POISON.

You should be shocked to learn what is in your municipal water supply and who controls it as well. Many local municipal water companies are foreign-owned companies, such as Veolia North America, a French owned company. Why this national security issue regarding one of our most important resources is accepted is a very big concern. You can get a report of what is in your water by requesting a copy of the "Consumer Confidence Report" from your water company, updated each year by early July.

A better source of information can be obtained from the Environmental Work Group (EWG.org). You can go on their website and find a better standard and more in-depth list of what contaminants are in your local water. This is a better resource as they do more testing and have more up-to-date information about probable toxic chemicals in our water, as our government water standards have not been updated for twenty years.

Water filtration can remove many of these contaminants, but fluorine is one of the hardest to get out. A good reverse osmosis system in your home can eliminate a majority of the toxins in drinking water and a carbon filter on your shower head can be beneficial as well so you are not absorbing these toxins through your skin.

FLUORIDE

Fluoride is not only ineffective but is also toxic by-product of the aluminum industry. It is a hazard to humans, animals and the environment. Fluoride was propagandized as a possible health treatment and then implemented after WWII. Before it was ingrained in our health system, it was a known environmental toxin and companies paid out many settlements for pollution because of it.

Possible side effects are low IQ in children, kidney disease, bone cancer, arthritis, dental and bone fluorosis, vascular illnesses and it is a possible carcinogen.

The following is a list of contaminants and the percentage found in my local water source, showing what exceeds EWG.org guidelines:

Chemical	Level	Hazard
Arsenic	720x	Carcinogen
Bromodichloromethane	41x	Carcinogen
Chloroform	68x	Carcinogen
Chromium (hexavalent)	21x	Carcinogen – what Erin Brockovich fought in her case
Dibromochloromethane	7.3x	Carcinogen
Haloacetic Acid (HAA5)	220x	Carcinogen
Haloacetic Acid (HAA9)	498x	Carcinogen
Total Trihalomethanes	192x	Carcinogen
Radium (both 226 & 228)	3.6x	Carcinogen
Tetrachloroethylene	3.7x	Carcinogen
Uranium	10x	Carcinogen

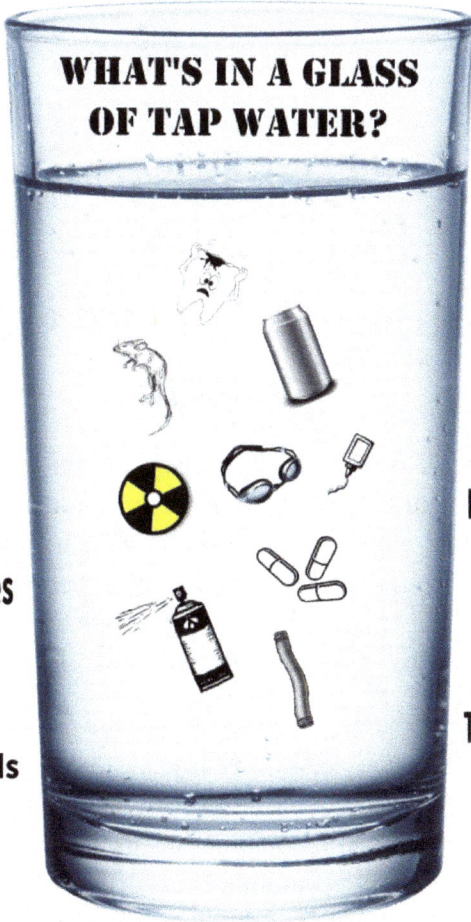

WHAT'S IN A GLASS OF TAP WATER?

Arsenic

Radioactive Contaminants

Pesticides

Nitrates

Hormones

Fluorine compounds

Calcium

Hexavalent Chromium

Lead

Pharmaceutical Drugs

Aluminium

Trihalomethanes (THMs)

(Source: www.bestwaterfilter.review)

- 12 -

CANCER HISTORY, LIES AND... IVERMECTIN?

A look at some of the history of cancer and its treatment in recent times brings out some very valuable information as the incidence of cancer has risen drastically in the US in the past 50 years. The US has one of the highest incidences of cancer per 100,000 people of any industrialized nation and is dramatically more than all undeveloped nations. We must ask why this is?

Almost all modern cancer treatments we have are biological warfare leftovers of WWI and WWII. Many of the pioneers of "cancer research" had Germanic names and it is easy to surmise that many of these "pioneers" came to America as a result of "Operation Paperclip". This brings up the question of what happened to all of the information about Nazi Germany's medical experimentation programs on holocaust victims—where did it go and who has it?

One of the most depraved individuals was Dr. Cornelius Rhoads, also known as the father of modern cancer treatment. Dr. Rhoads was in charge of military chemical and biological warfare, had a seat on the atomic energy commission, was the vice president of the American Cancer Society and the director of the Sloan Kettering Cancer Center. He also was a racist who performed horrific experiments on our own citizens, members of the military (60,000 members), targeted African Americans, Japanese Americans and Puerto Ricans, leaving a wake of those dead or suffering lifelong debilitations. He also infected Puerto Rican citizens with cancer, "coincidentally" at the same time a parasitic hookworm and tropical sprue took over the island. Here is an excerpt from a letter sent by Dr. Cornelius Rhoads:

> I can get a damn fine job here and am tempted to take it. It would be ideal except for the Porto Ricans. They are beyond doubt the dirtiest, laziest, most degenerate and thievish race of men ever inhabiting this sphere. It makes you sick to inhabit the same island with them. They are even lower than Italians. What the island needs is not public health work but a tidal wave or something to totally exterminate the population. It might then be livable. I have done my best to further the process of extermination by killing off 8 and transplanting cancer into several more. The latter has not resulted in any fatalities so far... The matter of consideration for the patients' welfare plays no role here — in fact all physicians take delight in the abuse and torture of the unfortunate subjects.

(Source: www.gizmodo.com/the-horrifying-letter-in-which-a-scientist-confessed-1507897479)

In addition to statements like this, the following is from the American Association of Cancer Research "Although gases were not used on the battlefield in World War II..., a great deal of research was done on vesicant war gases. The experience in WWI and the effects of an accidental spill of sulfur mustards on troops from a bombed ship in Bari Harbor, Italy, in WWII led to the observation that both bone marrow and lymph nodes were markedly depleted in those men exposed to the mustard gas."

(Source: aacrjournals.org/cancerres/article/6 8/21/8643/541799/A-History-of-Cancer-Chemotherapy)

If a victim of cancer treatment survives five years, the medical field considers that a "cure" as 97% of patients die within five years. A disproportionate 30-40% develop chemotherapy-induced peripheral neuropathy. Chemotherapy is only 3% effective and many patients develop and then die from radiation-induced necrosis (death of tissue) of the brain and vital organs. Chemotherapy has three classes of so-called drugs: alkylating agents, antimetabolites and antitumor antibiotics. These chemotherapy agents contain:

- **Alkylating Agents:** in this case, *mustard gas*; nitrogen mustards, thiotepa, bisulfan, nitrosoureas, mitomycin, procarbazine, dacarbazine.
- **Taxanes:** paclitaxel, docetaxel, nab-paclitaxel
- **Topoisomerase II inhibitors:** etoposide
- **Platinum (metal) Complexes:** Cisplatin, carboplatin, oxyplatin
- **Anthacylines:** doxorubicin, daunorubicin, idarubicin, mitoxantrone
- **Antimetabolites:** methotrexate, purine antagonists
- **Tubulin interactive agents:** vincristine, vinblastine
- **Miscellaneous agents:** bleomycin, asparaginase, hydroxyurea

These agents are extremely toxic and are themselves carcinogens designed to cause nuclear and mitochondrial DNA damage. They are demyelinating so they strip the nerves of their protective sheaths, causing neuropathy, ataxia, myokymia, optic neuropathy, Lhermitte's phenomenon, mimicking Guillain-Barré syndrome with myelopathy and a whole host of other serious conditions and, of course, very often, death.

PARASITES?

Would it be a surprise to you that most what is called "cancer" could possibly be simply a parasitic infestation? Parasites come in many forms such as protozoa, helminths, ectoparasites and intracellular parasites. Once again, you must recognize our enemy—the big pharma companies profit from our *illness*es. If they can hype cancer as some nebulous disease that can strike anyone, anytime and that you must act immediately without question or your own research, they will do it! They do this *every* day to thousands of Americans. They use the fear of death as their main weapon to enrich themselves without regard to how their victims fare.

Here is an eye-opening activity: do an internet search for "cancer cell" and it will bring up loads of computer-generated images, cartoons and animations but not a single image of an actual cancer cell. Now search "cancer histology" and "cancer endoscopy" and you will find some actual images of cancer "tumors and cells". Then search "bovine parasite endoscopy and histology" and you will find some similar images. Nobody speaks about parasitic infestations in America any longer, but our livestock are often infested with parasites that attack from hoof to head and many parasites are alive and well in our house pets!

Depending on the parasite, the infestation manifests in different ways. Our bodies will form large cysts or sacks to isolate the infestation to a local area. When the doctors do a biopsy, they puncture the protective sack our bodies created and this causes the "cancer" (or parasitic infection) to break out and spread all over.

One such parasite, Toxoplasma gondii, is spread by household and feral cats. It may cause slight flu-like symptoms and leave cysts in your body for decades. This can cause behavioral and psychological problems, the backstory for the saying "crazy cat lazy".

Breast cancer could be parasitic cysts or even just calcified ducts! The same could go for the numerous digestive tract cancers and cancers of other vital organs such as the pancreas, liver and brain. Parasites of the digestive tract have been plaguing humans for thousands of years—why would we think they just stopped using us a host in the past fifty or more years?

Some doctors say that certain types of cancers are intracellular parasites and this makes very good sense on many levels if you look at the images of many "cancers" compared to parasites. Additionally, there are many medical publications on PubMed and the NIH website that show the effectiveness of Avermectin parasitic drugs and its derivatives (ivermectin, selamectin, doramectin, eprinomectin and abamectin) at treating cancers of all types. Now you can see after the Covid plandemic why the establishment was so quick to discredit ivermectin and prevent you from using it.

One notable study on Pubmed.gov is PMC10054244 "Outcome of Ivermectin in cancer treatments: An experience in Loja-Ecuador". This study shows the effectiveness of IVM (ivermectin) as a cancer treatment and the associated dosage is in the following excerpt from this study:

> Likewise, another important aspect to consider is the dosage that people receive. Thus, according to the study results, the dose is directly related to weight rather than age. Usually, the dose ranges from 1–2 mL to 3–5 mL administered intramuscularly once or twice a month. Some indicated that they felt positive effects after IVM application, and others indicated that they felt side effects such as diarrhea, vomiting, stomach pain, etc.
>
> The IVM toxicity study in humans gives us a better idea of side effects. This study indicates that a dose between 0.05 and 0.40 mg/kg does not cause unwanted effects and risk to human life; doses between 6.6 and 8.6 mg/kg are toxic, causing vomiting, blurred vision, mydriasis, ataxia, tremor, and coma, and finally, lethal doses are of 24 mg/kg.

Source: Jiménez-Gaona Y, Vivanco-Galván O, Morales-Larreategui G, Cabrera-Bejarano A, Lakshminarayanan V. Outcome of Ivermectin in Cancer Treatment: An Experience in Loja-Ecuador. Nurs Rep. 2023 Feb 22;13(1):315-326. doi: 10.3390/nursrep13010030. PMID: 36976682; PMCID: PMC10054244.

This same study also concluded that people with epilepsy had a lower number of seizures after treatment with ivermectin.

Other studies on PubMed have shown the effectiveness of ivermectin, and other avermectin derivatives, inhibiting colorectal cancer cells, prostate cancer and ovarian cancer, inducing cytostatic autophagy in breast cancer, cervical cancer and more.

There is an additional antiparasitic drug called Fenbendazole and its class of drugs that I have seen many storys and videos of the person that was treated and cured of "cancer" after taking it. These stories range from terminal lung, brain cancer to bladder and colon. In each case they took the recommended dosage by body weight and were cured within a couple months leaving the experts confounded and the skeptics befuddled.

With all this information, you can see why the government is the gatekeeper of all cancer information, if cancer is indeed a parasitic infection (or some microorganism). This would also explain why the average person has cancer 6-10 times in their lifetime and do not know it. Additionally, 27% of people with cancer that do not do any treatment find the "cancer" disappears.

Finally, why does ingesting a mild toxic substance like mistletoe kill cancer cells? It is because we are the stronger organism so the mistletoe will not kill us but it will kill the parasites, just like avermectin drugs. In case you missed it, mistletoe is an approved cancer drug in many countries. Sulfa drugs (sulfonamide) also kill parasites and much more but they took this over-the-counter common cure off the shelves around the same time modern cancer treatments appeared after WWII.

Anecdotally, it seems that very few people die from "cancer"—they generally die from side effects of the "treatment." Modern treatments are generally as follows: puncture the protective sack, which causes a massive spread of the "cancer" (parasite), then cut out the "cancer" (surgery), then poison (chemotherapy) and then burn (radiation).

This lunacy can be illustrated by looking at your garden. Imagine you have one weed in the middle of your pristine garden. Instead of treating the problem you institute the cut-poison-burn method. You dig out the one weed with a backhoe, then spray poison on your entire garden. Then you proceed to use an industrial torch and burn everything. You do all of this in the hope that everything will return to a living and vibrant plot with no further weeds. If you have any garden experience, you will know that if you did this the only thing that would return is the weeds and they would come back with a vengeance and to the demise of any healthy seed you purposefully planted.

Most "cancer" is just an infestation that is caused by a compromised immune system. You have an injury, stress or severe emotional distress that weakens your system and the parasites take off. If you had dormant parasitic cysts, they activate in the weakened system and spread. You can see this in your own backyard with an injured fruit tree—once weakened, it is susceptible to parasitic borers and the tree is infested and begins to suffer and eventually die. If you forget to water your lawn for a few days in the summer heat, it browns a bit and that brown patch will soon be full of weeds. Our bodies respond much the same as these organisms.

The best advice until further research has been done is to not do early "cancer screening" as many people are misdiagnosed, and many "tumors" will remain static or even go away on their own. A Canadian study showed that women who had routine mammograms had a 52% increase in breast cancer diagnoses. A National Cancer Institute (NCI) study suggests that mammograms cause more cases of breast cancer than they identify.

A 1994 study showed that chemotherapy is 97% ineffective, meaning it only works 3% of the time. So why do cancer doctors continue to use it? Would you trust a car with brakes that worked 3% of the time? Cancer is big business and chemotherapy is the ONLY class of drugs that the prescribing doctor receives a direct portion from the sale of the cancer drugs and treatments. The following charts show the exponential rise in cancer treatment costs and the greed associated with them. The treatments have not changed, manufacturing of the drugs has not changed, so why has the price increased dramatically year over year?

Average Annual Costs For Oncology Products by Launch Year in the United States

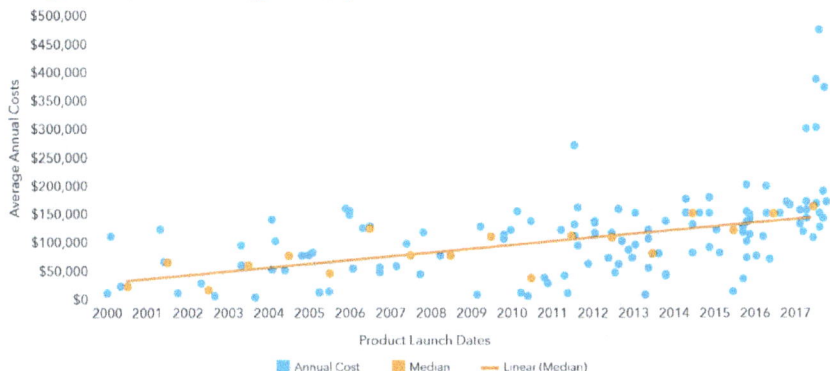

Source: IQVIA Institute, Apr 2018

Notes: If published annual costs are available they have been included, and if not, annual costs were estimated based on IQVIA Institute interpretation of the most-common dosing in the approved label and available product unit pricing information.

Report: Global Oncology Trends 2018: Innovation, Expansion and Disruption. IQVIA Institute for Human Data Science, May 2018

The cost of cancer drugs is soaring

Price at time of FDA approval in 2014 dollars

- Individual drugs monthly   Montly median price 5 years

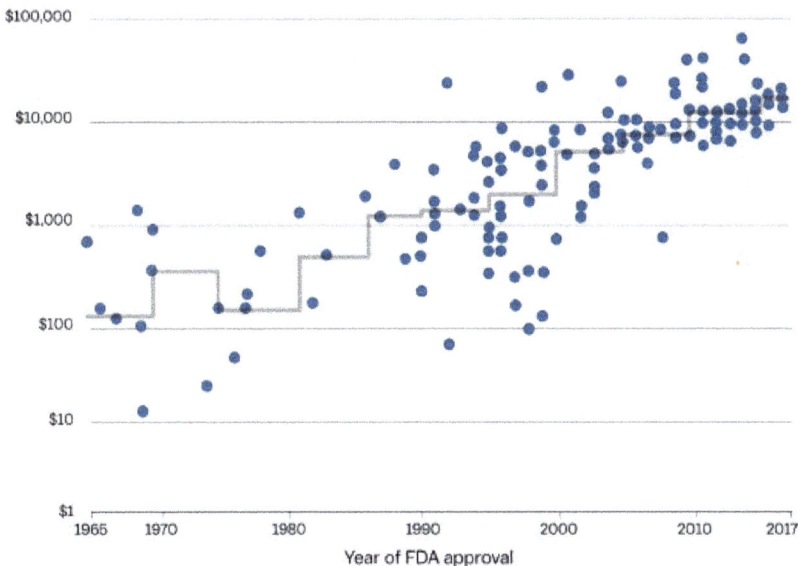

Source: Peter B. Bach, MD, Memorial Sloan Kettering Cancer Center

Vox

Remember that, as of 2016, over 12 million Americans have a misdiagnosed illness every year. A contrasting MRI is not necessary and the chemicals used are toxic and cumulative heavy metals (gadolinium, iron, platinum) will cause you much worse issues in other ways. This just gives the medical system an opportunity to double bill your insurance and further poison you with toxic metals.

If you have seen anyone go through cancer treatment, they do not die from cancer but from the treatment itself, and the ones that survived the treatment are left impaired, maimed, sterile, etc. A cancer patient's body is loaded with toxic metals and chemicals, immunocompromised and vulnerable to more attacks from parasites, other diseases and the effects of heavy metals.

Modern cancer treatment is barbaric, cruel and a satanically greed-driven system using a campaign of fear, lies and terror. There are certainly cases of cancer that are not parasitic infections as seen from exposure to chemicals or even severe injuries. These need specific treatments as well but will still not need toxic chemotherapy or radiation.

If you have "cancer," there are hundreds of possible remedies as "cancer" takes years or even longer to develop. Do not succumb to the "you have two weeks to live" line and do not let them use fear to control your actions. Take a step back, pray and do some research; take control of your own health by researching alternative medicines, treatments and healthcare providers.

These revelations again highlight some of the nefarious nature of the Covid-19 vaccine. You have to ask yourself why does an antiparasitic drug effectively neutralize the Covid-19 "virus"? The Covid-19 virus is clearly an engineered bioweapon and the "cure" (vaccine) is an engineered bioweapon created to depopulate the world. Are the huge blood clots found in Covid-19 vaccination victims a genetically modified parasitic organism? We do not have answers to this question yet but it is intriguing given the information coming to light. This would also explain why the Covid vaccine victims have "turbo cancer". Only time will tell what has been done in the dark and supplanted on the American population.

There has to be a better way to look at "cancer" and its treatment. Our health care system and our government clearly has not provided any better outcomes, treatments or preventative measures and once again, we must take our health back into our own hands and not blindly trust the system.

The Dollar Cost of Cancer

A look at cancer by the numbers from the American Grandparents Association

In the U.S., men have a **1** in **2** risk and women have a **1** in **3** **risk of developing** cancer during their lifetimes.

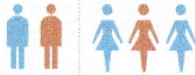

The **medical costs** of cancer care are $125 billion, with a projected increase to $158 billion by 2020.

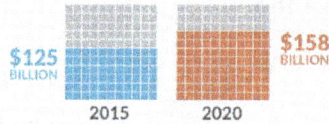

$125 BILLION — 2015

$158 BILLION — 2020

Lost productivity due to cancer is estimated to increase from $115.8 billion in 2000 to $147.6 billion in 2020.

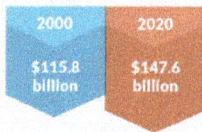

2000 — $115.8 billion
2020 — $147.6 billion

20% of cancer patients spend their entire **life savings** to get cancer care.

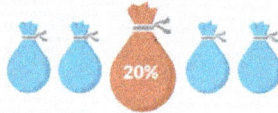

Newly approved **cancer drugs** now cost an average of $10,000 per month, with some exceeding $30,000 per month.

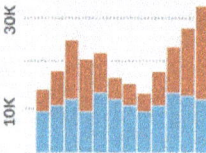

30K
10K

8 Most Expensive Cancers:
(in order of highest to lowest **annual cost** for the first year of treatment)

Cancer	Men	Women
Brain	$115,250	$108,168
Pancreatic	$94,092	$93,462
Ovarian		$82,324
Esophageal	$79,822	$79,532
Stomach	$78,453	$71,076
Lung	$60,885	$60,533
Lymphoma	$60,701	$57,881
Colorectal	$51,812	$51,327

In 2003, 1 in 10 privately insured cancer patients reported spending more than $18,585 (that's $24,104 in 2015 dollars!) **out of pocket** on care.

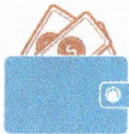

Statistics gathered from: American Cancer Society's Cancer Facts & Figures 2015 report; American Society of Clinical Oncology; American Association for Cancer Research; National Cancer Institute; Health Affairs.

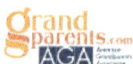

grandparents.com AGA — The American Grandparents Association connects, educates, and engages America's 70 million grandparents and their families by offering information, benefits, and discounts on healthcare, travel & more. Visit us at grandparents.com.

- 13 -

VACCINES: ENJOY YOUR MERCURY, ALUMINUM & A PINCH OF ABORTED HUMAN FETAL CELLS

Vaccines have become a very hot topic in the last several decades but especially since the Covid- 19 vaccine assault appeared on the horizon. Personally, I can say definitively that the foundation of my personal health problems began with the accumulation of over four dozen vaccines received in the military.

Vaccines, in conjunction with mercury-filled dental amalgams, innocuously called "silver fillings", led me down a miserable path of chronic illness, depression, anxiety, fibromyalgia, Hashimoto's thyroiditis, kidney stones, "mad hatter's" syndrome and more. It is also my opinion that vaccines, in combination with Bt-ridden GMO foods, cause autism and a long list of other diseases and chronic illnesses, often starting in childhood.

In the GMO section of this book, this idea was explored more in-depth, but the basics are that Bt GMO's cause leaky gut so when you get a vaccine, your body tries to remove the mercury, aluminum, formaldehyde, etc. through urine and feces but the leaky gut allows the toxins to pass directly into the blood stream and abdominal cavity, causing an immune response. This is the reason why, when administered from birth through the first few months and years of life, so many babies and toddlers—who almost certainly already have leaky gut from birth—have seizures, fever, paralysis, gastrointestinal problems and even personality changes, all of which eventually lead to autism diagnoses.

In the chapter on mercury that follows, I cover the chelation therapy that may strongly benefit those suffering from autism, multiple sclerosis, Parkinson's disease, and other topics presented in the back of this book. Please read all the precautions related to chelation therapy and stick with the Andrew Cutler protocol. Do your research on the rest but adhere to his warnings and recommendations. This therapy has been effective for this author personally.

Heavy metal toxicity is, in my opinion, the missing puzzle piece for almost all major disease and chronic illness. Mercury, aluminum, lead, titanium, bismuth, arsenic, antimony and uranium are in our food, medicines, dental fillings, water and much more. Mercury is the most potent neurotoxin there is, besides manmade plutonium. Almost every vaccine that goes into humans and livestock contains mercury (referred to as "thimerosal" in ingredient lists). No vaccines have ever been proven to be safe or effective. Vaccines contain the DNA and/or RNA of a live virus and many now include a totally new and unproven mRNA addition. There are also a number of toxins added into the vaccines as fillers and preservatives (called "adjuvants").

Vaccines are so dangerous that the manufacturers petitioned President Reagan telling him they would have to start discontinuing vaccine production because of the inherent dangers that would cost the companies greatly. In a horrible move, President Reagan obliged and signed a bill that absolved vaccine manufacturers from any liability claims from then on. President Reagan, in another misleading bill, allowed government employees to patent and benefit from patents of pharmaceuticals and treatments, fueling their greed more while simultaneously stifling the advancement of innovative and helpful cures.

AUTISM SIDEBAR

As we have repeatedly seen, our government and big pharma do not have our best interest in mind. Look at the programming the government and media do in coordination. Remember the 1988 movie *Rain Man* that premiered, to great accolades, at a time when "autism" was relatively unheard of? The movie portrayed Dustin Hoffman as an "idiot savant" with a gift in mathematical calculations. For many of us, this was our first introduction to "autism". The term "idiot savant" has been sidelined but the idea of autism took root and grew into the "spectrum" we constantly hear of today.

Everything you see on TV is for one purpose, it is called "programming" because the government, in cooperation with the media, are conditioning you to the trends, ideas, fears and topics *they* want you to focus on. We were being conditioned to the idea of autism because two years earlier, in 1986, President Reagan signed the National Childhood Vaccine Injury Act (NCVIA) that eliminated financial liability of vaccine makers due to vaccine injury claims.

Now look at the vaccine schedule changes from the 1970's when they added the MMR (Measles, Mumps, Rubella) vaccine. This coincides with every autism timeline chart available—all of them start at 1970. The vaccine schedule was updated in 1989, interestingly, the year after the Rain Man movie was released. The schedule was updated again in 1994-95 to add the Hep B vaccine, which is for a sexually transmitted disease and is not necessary for infants. Coincidentally, 1994 was the same year Bt GMO's were introduced into the food chain and, perhaps, not surprisingly, from 1994 on the cases of autism explode. The year 1999 shows an even bigger jump in autism with the addition of new Varicella and Rotavirus vaccines being added along with Hep A in 2000.

It is my opinion that mercury from vaccines and amalgam fillings and aluminum from vaccines and other consumable products may be the underlying cause of a huge list of diseases such as:

- Allergies
- Asthma

- Autoimmune Diseases
- Amyotrophic Lateral Sclerosis (ALS or Lou Gehrig's Disease)
- Ankylosing Spondylitis
- Myasthenia Graves
- Parkinson's Disease
- Hashimoto's Thyroiditis
- Hyper-parathyroiditis
- Hypothyroidism
- Schizophrenia Spectrum Disorders
- Anxiety
- Panic Attacks
- Personality Disorders
- ADHD
- Autism
- Depression
- Endocrine Disorders
- OCD
- Manic Depression
- Rheumatoid Arthritis
- Osteoarthritis
- Lupus Erythematosus
- Hypersensitivity to Light, Sound and/or Chemicals
- Chronic Fatigue
- Fibromyalgia
- Sciatica
- Gastritis
- IBS
- Sleep Paralysis
- Colitis
- Crohn's Disease
- Anorexia
- Bulimia
- Tremors

- Seizures
- Multiple Sclerosis
- Unprovoked Suicidal Thoughts
- Scleroderma
- High/Low Blood Pressure
- Brain Fog

I personally know this list very well as I have experienced a host of these issues and illnesses myself. Many of them were immediately relieved with the removal of my dental amalgams but, unfortunately, mercury is cumulative, and some widespread damage was incurred over the decades of exposure. I also have a very personal vendetta against this crime of mercury poisoning as I believe it claimed my mother with "Parkinsonoid" disease.

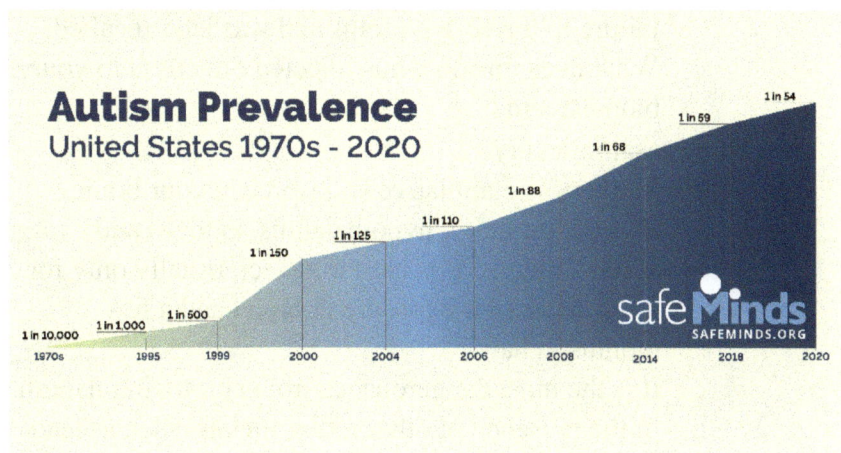

Here is a list of some of the preservatives (adjuvants) and ingredients they put in vaccines:

- Ammonium sulphate: known to cause liver and kidney damage and gastrointestinal damage
- Aluminum phosphate: linked to Alzheimer's
- Ammonium hydroxide: linked to Alzheimer's
- Amphotericin B: damages urinary tract, bowels and heart function
- Fetal embryo cells: two human cell lines taken from

aborted babies in the 1960's
- Formalin: or formaldehyde; known carcinogen and embalming fluid
- Fetal bovine serum: from cow calves; transmitter of mad cow disease
- Human diploid cells: from aborted baby fetal tissue
- Monosodium Glutamate or MSG: known carcinogen, linked to obesity
- Phenol red: toxic dye, linked to kidney, liver, respiratory and heart damage.
- Phenoxyethanol: a neurotoxin
  - In 2008, a nipple cream containing phenoxyethanol was on the market that caused gastrointestinal distress and nervous system depression as well as failure to thrive symptoms and was later recalled.
  - What does this do when injected directly into your bloodstream?
- Thimerosal: mercury;
  - Mercury is cumulative and stores in your brain, thyroid, pituitary, hypothalamus, kidneys and adrenal glands. It is hard to detect, usually only for a few days after exposure in blood and a few months in hair.
  - It is the most dangerous natural neurotoxin on earth.
  - In the presence of other heavy metals, such as lead and cadmium, mercury's effects are 100x.

Again, in my opinion, mercury, in conjunction with Bt GMO food products that cause leaky gut, vaccines are the underlying cause of autism and most chronic illness, ranging from Parkinson's to fibromyalgia to kidney disease and even birth defects.

Thimerosal has now been removed from childhood vaccines but, the flu, tetanus and any multi-dose vial vaccine still has mercury.

Single dose vials are sometimes free from mercury, but many doctors will still give children doses from adult multidose vials because it saves money (you get ten doses for the price of one).

If you absolutely must get vaccinated, make sure you physically see the vial they draw from and read the label and write down the lot and serial number.

Mercury causes severe inflammation and cell death. Period.

YEAR	VACCINE	YEAR	VACCINE
1914	Pertussis	1996	Hepatitis A
1926	Diphtheria	1998	Rotavirus - removed from market in 1999
1938	Tetanus	2000	Pneumococcal conjugate
1945	Inactivated Influenza	2003	Intranasal Influenza
1948	Diphtheria Tetanus & Pertussis (DTP)	2005	Meningococcal ACWY conjugate
1955	Inactivated Polio (shot)	2005	TDaP for adolescents
1962	Live Polio (oral)	2006	HPV for adolescent girls
1963	Measles	2006	Rotavirus
1967	Mumps	2009	HPV for adolescent boys
1969	Rubella	2013	Inactivated and intranasal Influenza
1971	MMR - same time autism charting begins	2014	Meningococcal B
1981	Hepatitis B	2014	HPV - for 9 types
1985	Hib	2017	Shingles
1992	DTaP	2017	Hepatitis B for adults
1995	Varicella		

On YouTube you can find a video showing an aluminum-mercury reaction. You can see a massive, expansive, exothermic chemical reaction. Just imagine if that reaction is happening, even on a microscopic level, to your brain cells or those of a newborn.

Below: Mercury and aluminum chemical reaction. One drop of mercury on an aluminum plate.

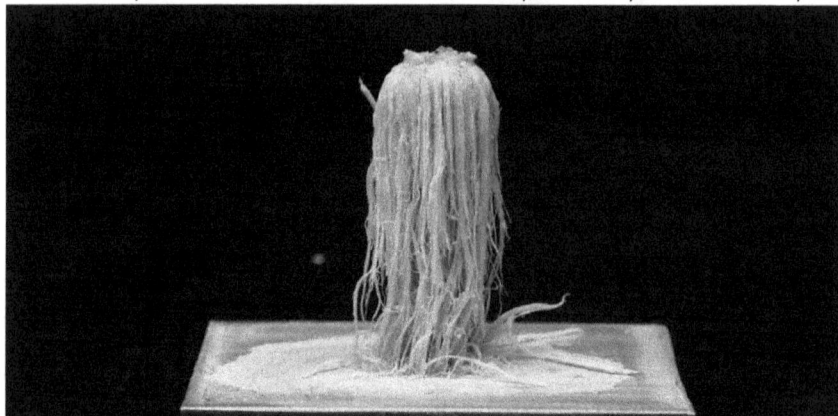

(Source: https://mobygeek.com/features/what-happens-when-mercury-meets-aluminum-1562)

In the last several years, we have seen the governmental tyrants around the globe force an experimental mRNA vaccine on the public through a fear campaign. Why was a vaccine even necessary when the original Covid-19 virus has a 99.889% survivability rate, the other variants an even higher rate? These mRNA vaccines have not been studied long enough, therefore being injected with this biologic toxin has been a massive crime against humanity, why else would the pharmaceutical companies want the records sealed for over 75 years?

Outside of the medical malpractice due to the overturn of routine protocols in the first years of the Covid pandemic, very few people succumbed to the actual virus. But after a year of the new mRNA vaccine implementation, the term "died suddenly" has become a new catch phrase in the news and media. Dying suddenly and unexpectedly has never been a trend but now we see this on a daily basis—almost always with a common background of having gotten this new vaccine.

The coroner's report of the dead shows massive blood clots—clots no one in mortuary science or forensics has ever seen before. We have seen young celebrities succumb to strokes or show up with Bell's Palsy and there are countless news stories about young, healthy athletes dropping dead.

As of 2023, there has been a:

- 279% spike in miscarriages
- 487% spike in breast cancer
- 551% spike in Guillain-Barre Syndrome
- 269% spike in Bell's Palsy
- 437% spike in ovarian dysfunction
- 680% Multiple Sclerosis

(Source: twitter @DrLoupis @diedsuddenly)

Look at the key players in the mRNA vaccine production and their push on the population and see what their motives are. Through fear, they gained power and took away freedom, which gives them more power. They killed millions with ventilators and vaccines and time will only tell how many more will die as a result of the medical malpractice thrusted on society.

Look at a few of the patents for Covid-19—the virus itself is patented—look at the names of the patent holders. They likely made a fortune off of our suffering. It is almost as if they knew this "pandemic" was coming as the virus and vaccine patents pre-dates 2020. These patents ensure the rights to the disease, the virus and detection methods for the virus, as well as biometrics methods for tracking, and all were patented and ready to go years before 2019. See the patent pages at the end of this chapter.

There is an excellent autism slideshow presented by AShotOfTruth.org, the following slides are just a couple highlights:

(Source: www.slideshare.net/ashotoftruth/a-shot-of-truth-thimerosal-timeline-33423446)

April 9, 2009

A new study in the journal Cellular Biology and Toxicology (Minami et al. 2010 Cell Biol Toxicol 26:143) showed that the induction of metallothionein (MT) messenger RNA (mRNA) and protein was observed in the cerebellum and cerebrum of mice after Thimerosal injection, as MT is an inducible protein. Metallothionein is a marker that would indicate the presence of mercury in these brain tissues as this study supports the possible biological plausibility for how low dose exposure to mercury from Thimerosal containing vaccines may be associated with autism.

2009: Not Your Typical Animal Testing

Rodrigues et al. reports that, in rat studies, "Of the total mercury found in the brain after TM exposure, 63% was in the form of Ino-Hg, with 13.5% as Et-Hg and 23.7% as Met-Hg." This affirms the previous work of Burbacher et al. (2005) on macaque monkeys where high levels of inorganic mercury, recalcitrant to excretion, accumulate and persist in brain tissues following Thimerosal exposure.

Dr. Ruth Etzel, USDA Division of Epidemiology and Risk Assessment, writes and to the American Academy of Pediatrics team involved with the July 7, 1999 public announcement. Dr. Etzel recommends a parallel path to the response of Johnson and Johnson to the 1982 outbreak of tainted Tylenol tablets: (1) act quickly to inform pediatricians that the products contain more Thimerosal (mercury) than we realized, (2) Be open with consumers as to why they didn't catch this earlier, and (3) show contrition. Dr. Etzel also alludes to the fact that despite these issues, the PHS will not show a preference to Thimerosal (mercury) free products.

VACCINE MERCURY BURDEN AND AUTISM RISK: UNITED STATES

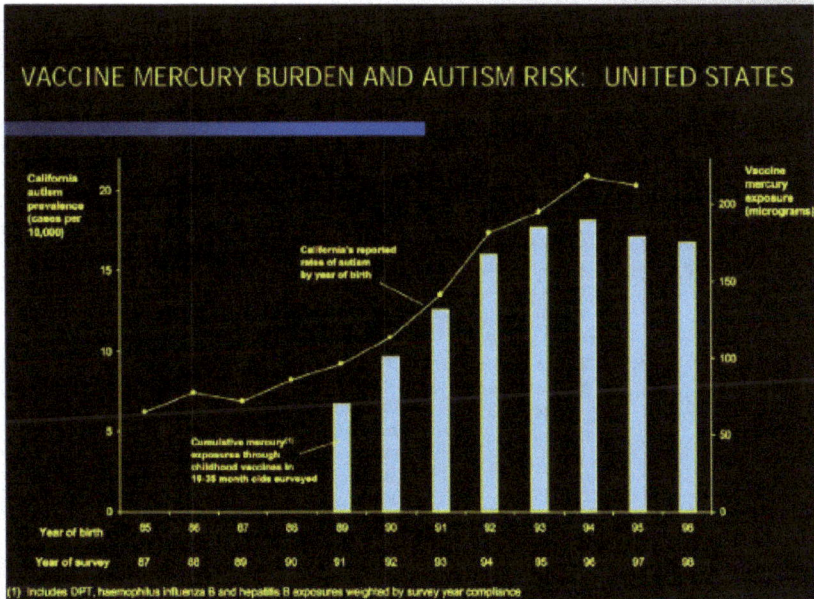

Vaccine Mercury Burden and Autism Risk Graph Source

1998: Autism Rate for Children Rising

Children are now receiving 237.5 mcg. of mercury from vaccines by age 18 months. According to a 2006 CDC report, the U.S. autism rate for children born in 1998 is 1 in 110.

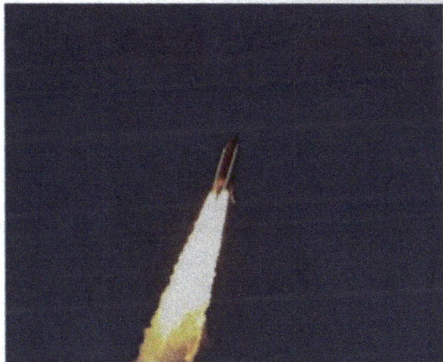

VACCINES DOSES for U.S. CHILDREN

1962   1983   2016

TOTAL DOSES: 5	TOTAL DOSES: 24	TOTAL DOSES: 72	
Polio	DTP (2 months)	Influenza (pregnancy)	Influenza (18 months)
Smallpox	OPV (2 months)	DTaP (pregnancy)	Hep A (18 months)
DTP	DTP (4 months)	Hep B (birth)	Influenza (30 months)
	OPV (4 months)	Hep B (2 months)	Influenza (42 months)
	DTP (6 months)	Rotavirus (2 months)	DTaP (4 years)
	MMR (15 months)	DTaP (2 months)	IPV (4 years)
	DTP (18 months)	HIB (2 months)	MMR (4 years)
	OPV (18 months)	PCV (2 months)	Varicella (4 years)
	DTP (4 years)	IPV (2 months)	Influenza (5 years)
	OPV (4 years)	Rotavirus (4 months)	Influenza (6 years)
	Td (15 years)	DTaP (4 months)	Influenza (7 years)
		HIB (4 months)	Influenza (8 years)
		PCV (4 months)	Influenza (9 years)
		IPV (4 months)	HPV (9 years)
		Hep B (6 months)	Influenza (10 years)
		Rotavirus (6 months)	HPV (10 years)
		DTaP (6 months)	Influenza (11 years)
		HIB (6 months)	HPV (11 years)
		PCV (6 months)	DTaP (12 years)
		IPV (6 months)	Influenza (12 years)
		Influenza (6 months)	Meningococcal (12 years)
		Influenza (7 months)	Influenza (13 years)
		HIB (12 months)	Influenza (14 years)
		PCV (12 months)	Influenza (15 years)
		MMR (12 months)	Influenza (16 years)
		Varicella (12 months)	Meningococcal (16 years)
		Hep A (12 months)	Influenza (17 years)
		DTaP (18 months)	Influenza (18 years)

*In 1986, Pharmaceutical manufacturers producing vaccines were freed from ALL liability resulting from vaccine injury or death by the Childhood Vaccine Injury Act.

With this, vaccines became HIGHLY profitable. There are 271 vaccines in development and mandatory vaccine laws for children — and ADULTS — being pushed in most states.

The US gives 2-3x more vaccines to children than most developed countries, yet we have some of the highest rates of childhood issues that are NOT seen in other countries. Things like asthma, childhood diabetes, food allergies, childhood leukemia, developmental delays, tics, ADHD, autism, lupus, arthritis, eczema, epilepsy, Alzheimers, brain damage, etc... **It's NOT a coincidence.**

Vaccines contain toxic chemicals that do NOT belong in our bodies, such as aluminum (known to cause brain and developmental damage even in small doses) and formaldehyde (known to cause cancer in humans).

LEARN THE RISK.ORG

VACCINE FACTS FROM AVoiceForChoice.org

If you are a parent who follows the CDC's VACCINE schedule, here are 20 FACTS you need to know to make an informed decision: Giving issues a voice, A Voice for Choice advocates for people's rights to be fully informed about the composition, quality, and short- and long-term health effects of all products that go into people's bodies, such as food, water, air, pharmaceuticals and cosmetics.

1. Vaccine manufacturers have NO liability (National Childhood Vaccine Injury Act of 1986), so CANNOT be sued for injury from their product and they have no incentive to make their product as safe as possible.

2. Vaccines are not held to the same double blind gold standard of clinical testing as other pharmaceutical drugs because they are considered biological products under the Public Health Federal Food, Drug and Cosmetic Act. They meet the same standards as cosmetics.

3. The per vaccine Federal Excise Tax is used to pay the vaccine injured through the government-created National Vaccine Injury Compensation Program (NVICP). $3.1 Billion has been paid to date (through 2015).

4. Vaccines contain neurotoxins (aluminum and mercury) far exceeding "safe levels" deemed by the EPA.

5. Vaccines contain cancer-causing ingredients, and have never been tested if they cause cancer, infertility or DNA mutation (Section 13.1 of every vaccine package insert).

6. Some vaccines are made from aborted fetal cell lines. (WI-38 and MC5-5 Human Cell Fibroblasts)

7. Vaccines are not 100% effective, and a vaccinated person can get the disease they were vaccinated for.

8. A vaccinated person carries the disease they were vaccinated for, "shedding" it, for up to 6 weeks.

9. The concept of herd/community immunity cannot be achieved by vaccines because vaccines are NOT 100% effective. Unlike lifetime immunity afforded by disease, vaccine-induced immunity lasts 2-10 years.

10. Doctors receive financial rewards from insurance companies for having patients fully vaccinated (~$400 per patient). They are advised NOT to share all the risks, or the vaccine package inserts, so 100% informed choices cannot be made in a doctor's office when vaccinating.

11. Vaccine injury is under-reported. VAERS is the only way to officially report a vaccine injury and is tedious with no incentive for a doctor to fill it out.

12. Vaccine mandates (like SB277 and SB792 in CA) literally hand over new customers to pharmaceutical companies and remove rights to choose what is injected into a person's body.

13. Pharmaceutical companies spend up to 19 times more on advertising than they do on research.

14. Corporate mainstream media gets 70% of their advertising revenue from pharmaceutical companies.

15. Vaccine safety and efficacy research is not conducted by independent researchers and so is biased.

16. The full CDC recommended vaccine schedule has never been tested. Vaccinated children are the human experiment.

17. All vaccines can cause injury or death, and there is no way to tell who will have a reaction.

18. Most doctors receive 30 MINUTES on vaccine education (that they are safe, effective and a must) during their 8 YEARS in medical school.

19. If someone dies from a vaccine, their family will be awarded no more than $250,000. Most cases of vaccine injury are dismissed because doctors and vaccine manufacturers deny a causation link. The statutory time limit for filing a claim is only 2 years after death and 3 years from the time of vaccine injury.

20. The government plan "Healthy People 2020" has a goal to fully

vaccinate all children and adults by 2020. There are 217 new vaccines being created right now.

(Source: avoiceforchoice.org/issues/pharmaceuticals-and-vaccines/20-vaccine-facts/)

CONCLUSION

As you can see, we need to be diligent to vet as much as we can, within the boundaries of sanity, before we inject or ingest anything into our bodies. We cannot control everything, but we can be discerning and diligent. Check everything you can. There is an overwhelming number of medicines, foods, vitamins and supplements that contain everything from mercury, lead, aluminum, titanium and dicyanide to Viagra, methamphetamine, synthetic steroids and sibutramine. The FDA does not require supplement manufacturers to go through testing and the FDA only checks a few of the millions of supplements on the market.

For example, I recently checked some favorite supplements and found out they contain unacceptable amounts of lead, mercury and dicyanide. Some of my favorite candies from the Mexican market had high levels of lead, as did a favorite brand of paprika. The information is often out there, but if the manufacturer will not provide an assay or third-party testing results, do not use the product. If you cannot find the information you need, weigh your options as to if you really need that product or not. After researching and writing many companies, I believe that if the company will not tell you pertinent details, it is because they do not want the results out, which is very concerning.

US007776521B1

(12) **United States Patent**
Rota et al.

(10) **Patent No.:** US 7,776,521 B1
(45) **Date of Patent:** Aug. 17, 2010

(54) **CORONAVIRUS ISOLATED FROM HUMANS**

(75) Inventors: **Paul A. Rota**, Decatur, GA (US); **Larry J. Anderson**, Atlanta, GA (US); **William J. Bellini**, Lilburn, GA (US); **Michael D. Bowen**, Decatur, GA (US); **Cara Carthel Burns**, Avondale Estates, GA (US); **Raymond Campagnoli**, Decatur, GA (US); **Qi Chen**, Marietta, GA (US); **James A. Comer**, Decatur, GA (US); **Byron T. Cook**, Augusta, GA (US); **Shannon L. Emery**, Lusaka (ZM); **Dean D. Erdman**, Decatur, GA (US); **Cynthia S. Goldsmith**, Lilburn, GA (US); **Jeanette Guarner**, Decatur, GA (US); **Charles D. Humphrey**, Lilburn, GA (US); **Joseph P. Icenogle**, Atlanta, GA (US); **Thomas G. Ksiazek**, Lilburn, GA (US); **Richard F. Meyer**, Roswell, GA (US); **Stephan S. Monroe**, Decatur, GA (US); **William Allan Nix**, Bethlehem, GA (US); **M. Steven Oberste**, Lilburn, GA (US); **Christopher D. Paddock**, Atlanta, GA (US); **Teresa C. T. Peret**, Atlanta, GA (US); **Pierre E. Rollin**, Lilburn, GA (US); **Mark A. Pallansch**, Lilburn, GA (US); **Anthony Sanchez**, Lilburn, GA (US); **Wun~Ju Shieh**, Norcross, GA (US); **Suxiang Tong**, Alpharetta, GA (US); **Sherif R. Zaki**, Atlanta, GA (US)

(73) Assignee: **The United States of America as represented by the Secretary of the Department of Health and Human Services, Centers for Disease Control and Prevention**, Washington, DC (US)

(*) Notice: Subject to any disclaimer, the term of this patent is extended or adjusted under 35 U.S.C. 154(b) by 96 days.

(21) Appl. No.: **11/748,359**

(22) Filed: **May 14, 2007**

Related U.S. Application Data

(62) Division of application No. 10/822,904, filed on Apr. 12, 2004, now Pat. No. 7,220,852.

(60) Provisional application No. 60/465,927, filed on Apr. 25, 2003.

(56) **References Cited**

U.S. PATENT DOCUMENTS

2005/0181357 A1 * 8/2005 Peiris et al. 435/5

FOREIGN PATENT DOCUMENTS

WO WO 2004/092360 10/2004

OTHER PUBLICATIONS

Ksiazek et al (New England Journal of Medicine 348:1953-1966, published online Apr. 10, 2003).*
Gut et al (Journal of Virological Methods 77:37-46, 1999).*
Neilan et al (Nucleic Acids Research 25:2938-9, 1997).*
Peiris et al (Lancet, 361:1319-1325, published online Apr. 8, 2003).*
Genbank Accession No. AY274119.1 GI:29826276 (Apr. 14, 2003).*
SARS-associated Coronavirus. Genomic Sequence Availability. [online] [retrieved on Aug. 8, 2005]. Retrieved from the Internet <URL: http://www.bcgsc.ca/bioinfo/SARS>.*
"Update: Outbreak of Severe Acute Respiratory Syndrome—Worldwide, 2003," *MMWR Weekly* 52:241-248, 2003.
Emery et al., "Real-Time Reverse Transcription-Polymerase Chain Reaction Assay for SARS-Associated Coronavirus," *Emerg. Infect. Diseases* 10:311-316, 2004.
Goldsmith et al., "Ultrastructural Characterization of SARS Coronavirus," *Emerg. Infect. Diseases* 10:320-326, 2004.
Ksiazek et al., "A Novel Coronavirus Associated with Severe Acute Respiratory Syndrome," *N. Engl. J. Med.* 348:1953-1966, 2003.
Luo and Luo, "Initial SARS Coronavirus Genome Sequence Analysis Using a Bioinformatics Platform," *2nd Asia-Pacific Bioinformatics Conference (APBC2004)*, Dunedin, New Zealand, 2004.
Marra et al., "The Genome Sequence of the SARS-Associated Coronavirus," *Science* 300:1393-1404, 2003.
Supplementary Online Material for Marra et al., www.sciencemag.org/cgi/content/full/1085953/DC1, (2003).
Rota et al., "Characterization of a Novel Coronavirus Associated with Severe Acute Respiratory Syndrome," *Science* 300:1394-1399, 2003.
Supplementary Online Material for Rota et al., www.sciencemag.org/cgi/content/full/1085953/DC1, (2003).
GenBank Accession No. AY274119, Apr. 14, 2003.
GenBank Accession No. AY278741, Apr. 21, 2003.
GenBank Accession No. AY278554.1, Apr. 18, 2003.
GenBank Accession No. AY278491.1, Apr. 18, 2003.
GenBank Accession No. AY278487, Apr. 21, 2003.

* cited by examiner

Primary Examiner— Mary E Mosher
(74) *Attorney, Agent, or Firm*— Klarquist Sparkman, LLP

(57) **ABSTRACT**

Disclosed herein is a newly isolated human coronavirus (SARS-CoV), the causative agent of severe acute respiratory syndrome (SARS). Also provided are the nucleic acid

‖‖‖‖‖‖‖‖‖‖‖‖‖‖‖‖‖‖‖‖‖‖‖
US007776521B1

(12) **United States Patent**   (10) **Patent No.:**   **US 7,776,521 B1**
Rota et al.   (45) **Date of Patent:**   **Aug. 17, 2010**

(54) **CORONAVIRUS ISOLATED FROM HUMANS**

(75) Inventors: **Paul A. Rota**, Decatur, GA (US); **Larry J. Anderson**, Atlanta, GA (US); **William J. Bellini**, Lilburn, GA (US); **Michael D. Bowen**, Decatur, GA (US); **Cara Carthel Burns**, Avondale Estates, GA (US); **Raymond Campagnoli**, Decatur, GA (US); **Qi Chen**, Marietta, GA (US); **James A. Comer**, Decatur, GA (US); **Byron T. Cook**, Augusta, GA (US); **Shannon L. Emery**, Lusaka (ZM); **Dean D. Erdman**, Decatur, GA (US); **Cynthia S. Goldsmith**, Lilburn, GA (US); **Jeanette Guarner**, Decatur, GA (US); **Charles D. Humphrey**, Lilburn, GA (US); **Joseph P. Icenogle**, Atlanta, GA (US); **Thomas G. Ksiazek**, Lilburn, GA (US); **Richard F. Meyer**, Roswell, GA (US); **Stephan S. Monroe**, Decatur, GA (US); **William Allan Nix**, Bethlehem, GA (US); **M. Steven Oberste**, Lilburn, GA (US); **Christopher D. Paddock**, Atlanta, GA (US); **Teresa C. T. Peret**, Atlanta, GA (US); **Pierre E. Rollin**, Lilburn, GA (US); **Mark A. Pallansch**, Lilburn, GA (US); **Anthony Sanchez**, Norcross, GA (US); **Wun-Ju Shieh**, Alpharetta, GA (US); **Sherif R. Zaki**, Atlanta, GA (US)

(73) Assignee: **The United States of America as represented by the Secretary of the Department of Health and Human Services, Centers for Disease Control and Prevention**, Washington, DC (US)

(*) Notice: Subject to any disclaimer, the term of this patent is extended or adjusted under 35 U.S.C. 154(b) by 96 days.

(21) Appl. No.: **11/748,359**

(22) Filed: **May 14, 2007**

Related U.S. Application Data

(62) Division of application No. 10/822,904, filed on Apr. 12, 2004, now Pat. No. 7,220,852.

(60) Provisional application No. 60/465,927, filed on Apr. 25, 2003.

(51) Int. Cl.

(56) **References Cited**

U.S. PATENT DOCUMENTS

2005/0181357 A1 *   8/2005   Peiris et al. 435/5

FOREIGN PATENT DOCUMENTS

WO   WO 2004/092360   10/2004

OTHER PUBLICATIONS

Ksiazek et al (New England Journal of Medicine 348:1953-1966, published online Apr. 10, 2003).*
Gut et al (Journal of Virological Methods 77:37-46, 1999).*
Neilan et al (Nucleic Acids Research 25:2938-9, 1997).*
Peiris et al (Lancet, 361:1319-1325, published online Apr. 8, 2003).*
Genbank Accession No. AY274119.1 GI:29826276 (Apr. 14, 2003).*
SARS-associated Coronavirus. Genomic Sequence Availability. [online] [retrieved on Aug. 8, 2005]. Retrieved from the Internet <URL: http://www.bcgsc.ca/bioinfo/SARS>.*
"Update: Outbreak of Severe Acute Respiratory Syndrome—Worldwide, 2003," *MMWR Weekly* 52:241-248, 2003.
Emery et al., "Real-Time Reverse Transcription-Polymerase Chain Reaction Assay for SARS-Associated Coronavirus," *Emerg. Infect. Diseases* 10:311-316, 2004.
Goldsmith et al., "Ultrastructural Characterization of SARS Coronavirus," *Emerg. Infect. Diseases* 10:320-326, 2004.
Ksiazek et al., "A Novel Coronavirus Associated with Severe Acute Respiratory Syndrome," *N. Engl. J. Med.* 348:1953-1966, 2003.
Luo and Luo, "Initial SARS Coronavirus Genome Sequence Analysis Using a Bioinformatics Platform," *2nd Asia-Pacific Bioinformatics Conference (APBC 2004)*, Dunedin, New Zealand, 2004.
Marra et al., "The Genome Sequence of the SARS-Associated Coronavirus," *Science* 300:1393-1404, 2003.
Supplementary Online Material for Marra et al., www.sciencemag.org/cgi/content/full/1085953/DC1, (2003).
Rota et al., "Characterization of a Novel Coronavirus Associated with Severe Acute Respiratory Syndrome," *Science* 300:1394-1399, 2003.
Supplementary Online Material for Rota et al., www.sciencemag.org/cgi/content/full/1085953/DC1, (2003).
GenBank Accession No. AY274119, Apr. 14, 2003.
GenBank Accession No. AY278741, Apr. 21, 2003.
GenBank Accession No. AY278554.1, Apr. 18, 2003.
GenBank Accession No. AY278491.1, Apr. 18, 2003.
GenBank Accession No. AY278487, Apr. 21, 2003.

* cited by examiner

Primary Examiner—Mary E Mosher
(74) *Attorney, Agent, or Firm*—Klarquist Sparkman, LLP

(57)   **ABSTRACT**

Disclosed herein is a newly isolated human coronavirus (SARS-CoV), the causative agent of severe acute respiratory syndrome (SARS). Also provided are the nucleic acid

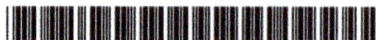

US007220852B1

(12) **United States Patent**
Rota et al.

(10) Patent No.: **US 7,220,852 B1**
(45) Date of Patent: **May 22, 2007**

(54) **CORONAVIRUS ISOLATED FROM HUMANS**

(75) Inventors: **Paul A. Rota**, Decatur, GA (US);
Larry J. Anderson, Atlanta, GA (US);
William J. Bellini, Lilburn, GA (US);
Cara Carthel Burns, Avondale Estates,
GA (US); **Raymond Campagnoli**,
Decatur, GA (US); **Qi Chen**, Marietta,
GA (US); **James A. Comer**, Decatur,
GA (US); **Shannon L. Emery**, Lusaka
(ZM); **Dean D. Erdman**, Decatur, GA
(US); **Cynthia S. Goldsmith**, Lilburn,
GA (US); **Charles D. Humphrey**,
Lilburn, GA (US); **Joseph P. Icenogle**,
Atlanta, GA (US); **Thomas G. Ksiazek**,
Lilburn, GA (US); **Stephan S. Monroe**,
Decatur, GA (US); **William Allan Nix**,
Bethlehem, GA (US); **M. Steven
Oberste**, Lilburn, GA (US); **Teresa C.
T. Peret**, Atlanta, GA (US); **Pierre E.
Rollin**, Lilburn, GA (US); **Mark A.
Pallansch**, Lilburn, GA (US); **Anthony
Sanchez**, Lilburn, GA (US); **Suxiang
Tong**, Alpharetta, GA (US); **Sherif R.
Zaki**, Atlanta, GA (US)

(73) Assignee: **The United States of America as
represented by the Secretary of the
Department of Health and Human**

FOREIGN PATENT DOCUMENTS

| WO | WO 2004/085633 | * 10/2004 |
| WO | WO 2004/092360 | * 10/2004 |

OTHER PUBLICATIONS

GenBank Accession No. AY274119, "SARS Coronavirus Tor2,
complete genome," version AY274119.1, Apr. 14, 2003.*
GenBank Accession No. AY278487, "SARS coronavirus BJ02,
partial genome," version AY278487.1, Apr. 21, 2003.*
Genbank Accession No. AY278554, "SARS coronavirus CUHK-
W1, complete genome," version AY278554.1, Apr. 18, 2003.*
GenBank Accession No. AY278491, "SARS Coronavirus HKU-
39849, complete genome," version AY278491.1, Apr. 18, 2003.*
SARS-associated Coronavirus. Genomic Sequence Availability.
[online] [retreived on Aug. 8. 2005]. Retreived from the Internet
<URL: http://www.bcgsc.ca/bioinfo/SARS>.*
GenBank Accession No. AY274119, Apr. 14, 2003.
GenBank Accession No. AY278741, Apr. 21, 2003.
"Update: Outbreak of Severe Acute Respiratory
Syndrome—Worldwide, 2003," *MMWR Weekly* 52:241-248 (2003).
Emery et al., "Real-Time Reverse Transcription-Polymerase Chain
Reaction Assay for SARS-Associated Coronavirus," *Emerg. Infect.
Diseases* 10:311-316 (2004).
Goldsmith et al., "Ultrastructural Characterization of SARS
Coronavirus," *Emerg. Infect. Diseases* 10:320-326 (2004).
Ksiazek et al., "A Novel Coronavirus Associated with Severe Acute
Respiratory Syndrome," *N. Eng. J. Med.* 348:1953-1966 (2003).
Luo and Luo, "Initial SARS Coronavirus Genome Sequence Analy-
sis Using a Bioinformatics Platform," *2nd Asia-Pacific Bioinformat-*

System and method for using, processing, and displaying biometric data

Publication Number: US-10910016-B2

Patent Family: US-10242713-B2; US-10522188-B2; US-10910016-B2; US-2017229149-A1; US-2019325914-A1; US-2020126593-A1;
US-2020381021-A1

Priority Date: 2015-10-13 Grant Date: 2021-02-02

Inventor(s): ROTHSCHILD RICHARD A; Macklin Dan; SLOMKOWSKI ROBIN S; HARNISCHFEGER TASKA

Assignee(s): ROTHSCHILD RICHARD A; Macklin Dan; SLOMKOWSKI ROBIN S; HARNISCHFEGER TASKA

Classification: G06K9/00; G11B27/031; G11B27/10; G16H40/63; G16H40/67; ...

Abstract: A method is provided for identifying and displaying video data of a user, either alone or together (in synchronization) with other data, such as biometric data acquired during a time that the video data was captured/received. The method includes storing biometric data separately from the video data, allowing the biometric data to be search quickly to identify at least one value (e.g., a value corresponding to at least one biometric event). At least one biometric time-stamp (e.g., a time, a sample rate, a position within a plurality of values, etc.) linked to the identified value can then be used to identify a corresponding video time-frame, which can then be used to play the video data, either alone or together with biometric data, starting at a particular time (e.g., at a time that the event occurred, shortly before the event occurred, etc.).

Linked Compounds Count: 1   Linked Substances Count: 1

System and method for testing for COVID-19

Publication Number: US-11024339-B2 **Patent Family:** US-11024339-B2; US-2020279585-A1; US-2021257004-A1

Priority Date: 2015-10-13 **Grant Date:** 2021-06-01

Inventor(s): ROTHSCHILD RICHARD A

Assignee(s): ROTHSCHILD RICHARD A

Classification: G06K9/00; G11B27/031; G11B27/10; G16H40/63; H04N5/76; ...

Abstract: A method is provided for acquiring and transmitting biometric data (e.g., vital signs) of a user, where the data is analyzed to determine whether the user is suffering from a viral infection, such as COVID-19. The method includes using a pulse oximeter to acquire at least pulse and blood oxygen saturation percentage, which is transmitted wirelessly to a smartphone. To ensure that the data is accurate, an accelerometer within the smartphone is used to measure movement of the smartphone and/or the user. Once accurate data is acquired, it is uploaded to the cloud (or host), where the data is used (alone or together with other vital signs) to determine whether the user is suffering from (or likely to suffer from) a viral infection, such as COVID-19. Depending on the specific requirements, the data, changes thereto, and/or the determination can be used to alert medical staff and take corresponding actions.

Linked Compounds Count: 1 **Linked Substances Count:** 1

- 14 -

DENTAL AMALGAM ILLNESS:
MAD HATTER'S SYNDROME
INSANE IN THE MEMBRANE

Have you ever heard of a medical quack? The term "quack" came from the German pronunciation for their word for mercury: "queck silber". We call it "quicksilver" for the same reason—because it moves as if it is alive. Back in the 1800's, the pioneers of dentistry were at odds with each other because of the mercury conflict. Some were saying that quicksilver (mercury) was dangerous, and they called the ones who wanted to use mercury "quacks". Like everything, the nomenclature has been distorted and perverted so that now the ones who go with the proven science are called "quacks".

Mad hatter disease, also called "mad hatter syndrome", refers to chronic mercury poisoning due to prolonged exposure to this toxic metal. It leads to severe neurological effects called "erethism". People who are repeatedly exposed to mercury are likely to develop mad hatter disease.

Do you have or know someone who has an unexplained illness that just appeared with sudden onset? Disorders such as anxiety, autism, long panic attacks, Parkinsonian-like symptoms, PTSD and/or Gulf War Syndrome, fibromyalgia, chronic fatigue, sciatica, chemical sensitivities, sensory overload, obsessive compulsive disorder, paranoia, anorexia, bulimia, arthritis, manic depressive disorder,

Hashimoto's thyroiditis, hypothyroidism, asthma, bruxism, allergies, mad hatters syndrome (erethism), sleep paralysis and more are linked to mercury and other heavy metal toxicity.

You may be shocked by the products that contain mercury and how many industries manufacture or produce things with it. It is used in vaccines (as thimerosal), dental amalgam (silver) fillings, some contact lens solutions, antifungal creams, medications and some supplements have trace amounts as well.

Mercury is widely used in the mining industry because when combined with other metals, such as gold, it adheres to the sought-after metal so that miners can process the precious metals. This also occurs in our bodies as mercury gobbles up selenium, which is vital for thyroid function. It almost certainly does this with a majority of other essential metals as well.

Dental amalgams contain 50% mercury by weight and they continuously off-gas every time you eat, drink hot liquids, brush your teeth or grind your teeth (incidentally, mercury causes bruxism). If you have a gold crown, it may have been set with amalgam and sometimes they even fill root canals with amalgam. If you have a gold tooth and amalgams you now have a worse situation because there is acid in saliva and now reactive metals so it is like having a battery in your mouth, causing more leeching of mercury. The amalgams also contain the toxic metals palladium, indium, as well as silver, zinc and copper.

If you have other heavy metals in your system (lead, cadmium, etc.), it makes mercury 100 times more damaging. Mercury is cumulative, storing in your brain, pituitary, hypothalamus, kidneys, adrenals and thyroid. It is hard to test unless you were recently exposed as the heavy metals hide deep in these vital organs—mercury hides in the brain—so there is not heavy metal coursing through your cardiovascular system or being excreted from the body.

This author purchased a mercury vapor analyzer and tested the amount of mercury vapor that was being emitted from his own amalgam fillings. After brushing one amalgam filling with a new toothbrush for 10 seconds, it was off-gassing at .105 mg/m^3. OSHA guidelines say that if a workplace measures .100 mg/m^3, operations should be shut down immediately and the company would be fined $10,000. Just the vapor coming from one tooth is a toxic environment according to OSHA standards!

It would seem that any measurable amount of mercury is toxic and its use is inexcusable and criminal. Untold millions of people are suffering from heavy metal toxicity from fillings, vaccines, foods and medicines. Our physical bodies operate as biological, electro-chemical machines and these heavy metals basically short circuit the system, causing severe inflammation. This inflammation from these toxins manifests themselves in every form of disease and autoimmune disease and chronic illness.

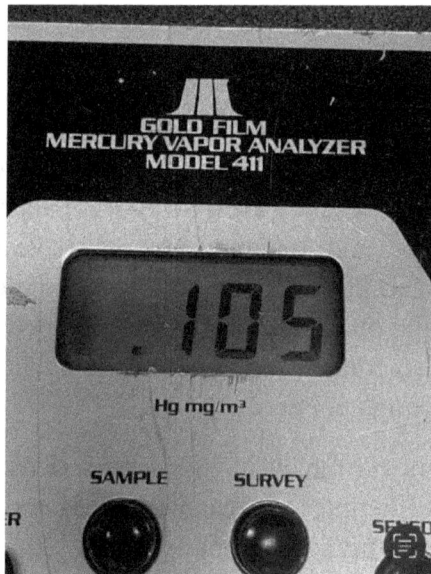

Author's own analysis results from one amalgam filled tooth in 2023.

This subject is very personal to me and this is where my exploration of the truth in food and medicine began. One day, over two decades ago, while still in the military, I had sleep paralysis after another round of vaccines, and from then on it would come and go along with cramps in my legs at night. A few years later I had a panic attack that lasted over a week with no sleep for days at a time. These became more progressive but still randomly occurring—as in there was not a trigger—from then on for over twenty years. I have been living in constant terror not knowing when it would strike again. None of this made sense either, as it did not meet the criteria for a "panic attack" since they are very short lived (15-30 minutes) and caused by stressors yet mine were random and could last for days.

After almost twenty years and a PTSD with anxiety disorder diagnosis, the panic attacks and anxiety was an everyday thing, not as intense but in a different form. Constant fear, paranoia, insomnia, frequent urination throughout the night, sciatica, fibromyalgia, allergies, sensitivity to sound/light/odors, depression and so on. I started searching for a pattern—what had happened recently to spiral my heath downward and what happened twenty years ago to trigger the first panic attack? The only thing I could think of in recent history was a few months before things went off the cliff for me physically and mentally was that I went to the dentist to repair a sizeable filling that fell out—an amalgam filling. Then I realized that I had had all my cavities fixed and paid for by the military about a month before the first attack twenty years ago. I did some research on dental anxiety and came across a video on YouTube called "smoking teeth" and "unbelievable healing story".

Thanks be to the Lord for this information because it has changed my life. Now I had the answer—the solution to the mystery. Twenty-five years ago, I had over four dozen vaccines, then twenty years ago I had over a dozen large mercury amalgams fillings put in. I then had acute mercury toxicity causing a massive panic event. Fast forward twenty years and I had my amalgam tooth drilled and filled without protections and was unknowingly exposed to another large amount of mercury causing a cascading autoimmune reaction.

My mother died from complications from early onset "Parkinson's disease," although looking back I think she also had heavy metal toxicity. She was exposed to heavy metals as an artist, she had multiple mercury amalgams and she had breast implants (which have platinum and other toxins). I say this because she had many "parkinsonism" traits but was missing some of the more notable ones like the writhing and uncontrollable shaking.

I believe I inherited a sensitivity to heavy metals from my mom, on top of some of it being passed from her to me in the womb—this is another way we accumulate heavy metals. I have to say it has been miserable, but God works out everything for my good and His glory. I can gladly say like the psalmist in Psalm 119:71: "It is good for me that I was afflicted, That I may learn Your statutes." God used this situation so that I would learn that I needed salvation, that I should humble myself before Him and repent of my sins and trust in Christ for everything so that my soul would be saved. This is the most important thing since this body is passing away and one day will die and then we will be moving from the temporal world to the eternal.

Because mercury is cumulative and can take decades to manifest its full damage, an individual outcome appears to be based on roughly a 20% genetics and 80% environmental toxins ratio. Your genetics will determine how the toxicity will manifest itself. If you take two people exposed to the same amount of mercury in vaccines one may get hypothyroidism and the other parkinsonism and someone else anxiety or schizophrenia. Other environmental factors obviously play a large role and will be very unique to each person.

Mercury from vaccines and dental amalgam fillings must be one of the most insidious, greedy and satanic things done to entire populations. If you think our government does not know they are poisoning us, just look at at all of the scandalous experiments our government has done to its citizens over the last few decades—just to name a few:

- Measles Vaccine Experiment
- Willowbrook Experiments
- Operation Big Buzz
- Operation Sea-Spray
- Operation Midnight Climax

- WWII Mustard Gas Experiments
- Plutonium Testing
- Navy Beef Blood Transfusions
- Stateville Penitentiary Malaria Study
- Tuskegee Syphilis Study
- MK Ultra
- Guatemalan STD Project
- PA Holmesburg Prison Agent Orange Experiments
- Infecting Puerto Rico with Cancer
- Project Artichoke
- US ARMY Germ Warfare Testing 1949-1969
- Operation Green Run
- Radioactive Iron Project
- Operation LAC
- Operation Top Hat
- Project CHATTER
- Project Bluebird
- Operation Crossroads
- Operation Dew
- Operation Whitecoat
- Project 112
- Covid-19 Vaccines

This is a list of just some of the testing that we know about though leaks, whistleblowers and court filings. They have not stopped these experiments—they are just better at hiding them in plain sight because we have been programmed and conditioned. Wicked men just get more wicked and each experiment gets more perverse. The more they see the populous as a threat to their power, the more desperate and depraved the globalist elites will become. The Covid Era should have taught us this: we were conditioned and programmed through fear and propaganda on every level, shamed into not researching or questioning any new rule, law or protocol. This is what they want—a sick, ignorant population that just obeys. A quiet, subdued population is not a threat to them, the thinkers are!

So be a thinker and take action.

We in the western world are circling the drain at an exponential rate, just as the Bible says in 2 Timothy 3:1-7:

> But realize this, that in the last days difficult times will come. For people will be lovers of self, lovers of money, boastful, arrogant, slanderers, disobedient to parents, ungrateful, unholy, unloving, irreconcilable, malicious gossips, without self-control, brutal, haters of good, treacherous, reckless, conceited, lovers of pleasure rather than lovers of God, holding to a form of godliness although they have denied its power; avoid such people as these. For among them are those who slip into households and captivate weak women weighed down with sins, led on by various impulses, always learning and never able to come to the knowledge of the truth.

MERCURY CONTAINING PRODUCTS TO BE AWARE OF:

Note: not all manufactures use thimerosal (mercury) or elemental mercury

Dental Amalgams (Silver Fillings)

Vaccines Human & Veterinary

Insecticides, Fungicides, Herbicides, Disinfectants

Vaginal Tablets, Douches, Creams

Hair Tonic (Mercuric Chloride)

Ammunition (Fulminated Mercury)

Veterinary Creams, Skin Treatments

Skin Whitener/Bleach Creams

Eye Drops, Contact Lens Solution

Paint & Tattoo Pigments

Latex, Acrylic, Oil Paint

Mildew, Mold Treatments

Fluorescent, Neon Lights, Vapor Lamp Bulbs

Nasal Sprays

Ear Drops

Psoriasis Creams

Fungal Creams

Antiseptics/First Aid Ointments/washes

Large Saltwater Fish

Some Supplements/Vitamins

Waterproof Mascara

Mercurial Diuretics

Antibiotics

Hemorrhoid Relief Ointment

- 15 -

PALLIATIVE CARE: ARE YOU OR A LOVED ONE A USELESS EATER?

Palliative comes from the Latin word "to cloak". Today it refers to a medical end-of-life and terminal illness care program that really started to take off in the late 1970's. This system of care is more or less the stage of care prior to a patient's death or prior to the move to hospice. Palliative care is for people with serious, chronic and/or long-term health problems such as cancer, dementia, Parkinson's Disease, COPD and other issues that the system has deemed "incurable." It provides a roadmap to how the patient wants their last days to unwind and removes drugs and equipment and eventually nutrition and hydration from the patient's regimen until all that is left are "comfort" care solutions (basically, opioids) to ease pain as death looms.

Palliative care got its biggest boost after the so-called Affordable Care Act of 2010. As more government regulation leaned on the medical system, costs rose, and protocols changed. The death models from Europe and Canada began to bubble to the surface in the US, labeled as "care". For instance, deaths specifically from Alzheimer's Disease rose 55% from 1999-2014, while from 2000-2011, hospitals with 50 or more palliative beds increased 157%, mostly after 2010.

FOLLOW THE MONEY

Researching palliative care reveals that physicians can bill insurance each time they just *talk* to a patient about end-of-life care. Medicare will also allow providers to bill a maximum of seven days of end-of-life care, billed in 15-minute increments.

One suspicious billing code for palliative care has to do with administering two vaccines (pneumococcal conjugate or polysaccharide vaccine) during end-of-life assessments. If palliative care requires stopping all medical treatments and just concentrating on comfort care why would they be concerned with a last-minute vaccine? Are they intentionally trying to make already-compromised patients sick from a vaccine? It would seem so since injecting toxins into someone who already has a compromised system with toxins will just make them worse.

The reason I personally started looking into this topic is because of my mother's Parkinsonism (which, as I said, I believe was actually undiagnosed heavy metal toxicity). In her final days, she cut her hand and went to the ER. She had no life-threatening symptoms and had not been in a particularly noticeable decline. She was still eating and drinking, talking, moving around and interacting with my dad. But the next thing you know, she went from a cut on her hand to being admitted to the hospital and within a few days, her system had "shut down" and she died. This similar situation happened with another family member and then another. The question in the back of my mind was always "how did she and the others die and so fast?" Their bodies and minds were functional in all cases but they died of a sudden system failure (renal, in my mother's case) and the rest of the body followed.

I found my answer while researching palliative care: my mother and the others had become useless eaters. The government and big pharma want us sick enough that they can make a profit from our misery and keep us dependent on them but when you become a burden it is lights out for you. *Shut up and die.*

Looking at the palliative care guidelines, the medical system classifies someone in one of three categories: stable, transitional or end-of-life. They have a questionnaire that the healthcare providers complete periodically during your stay and you are given a score. If you express discomfort, agree to DNR/DNI (do not resuscitate, do not intubate), if you agree to comfort care, if you have a serious condition, if are you dependent on care, these all flag you in the system.

If placed on palliative care you are given a code status of "Comfort Care Only" and they discontinue all orders and medication for treatment that are not for comfort, including discontinuing nutrition and IV hydration, deactivating implanted defibrillators and then remove and disconnect all monitors and silence room alarms (on monitors and the bed).

Next the provider chooses from morphine or fentanyl and administers it. This often gives the patient dyspnea, so they administer more opioids. If the patients become anxious from the dyspnea, they give some more opioids. Once agitation, restlessness or delirium sets in, they administer patients haloperidol. Other medications include lorazepam, prochlorperazine, ondansetron, metoclopramide, glycopyrrolate, hyoscyamine, scopolamine and ketorolac.

To break down the protocol simply, it goes like this:

- stop all treatment
- shut down all machines
- load the patient up on opioids/scopolamine
- the patient's body shuts down from lack of food and water (aka: acute renal failure)

This is what killed my mother, not Parkinsonism. The Affordable Care Act is just a soft euthanasia program, in line with the rest of the western world's system that are headed towards full communism.

In summary, if you want to be healthy, stay out of the hospitals, if at all possible, unless it is a true emergency (stroke, heart attack, car accident, etc.). This includes childbirth as it is not a medical condition or emergency and when you do it naturally everything is better—midwives are a fantastic option. Finally, if any medical personnel ask you about end-of-life care or for you to inject or ingest their poison tell THEM to shut up and die.

- 16 -

SAVE YOUR BODY: POSSIBLE TREATMENTS

Spiritual Conclusions

After everything we have been through in this book, I want to remind you to be a critical thinker, to examine all things, to take charge of your own health, education and life. Take the power back from the government, the education system and the healthcare system and stop rewarding them for poisoning us in every way possible. First make sure your soul is secure, then work on your body. You cannot control everything, so take control of what is reasonable and pray about the rest. Remember not to sit back and be passive in your life but to take charge.

Information and knowledge are power, so seek them while they may be found. Isaiah 55:6-7

> Seek Yahweh while He may be found;
> Call upon Him while He is near.
> Let the wicked forsake his way
> And the unrighteous man his thoughts;
> And let him return to Yahweh,
> And He will have compassion on him,
> And to our God,
> For He will abundantly pardon.

We are at war but not a conventional war with armies battling it out. It is a spiritual war where these demons use information, deception, mind-conditioning, propaganda and an all-out assault on the truth. They want us to be fat, sick and ignorant so they can maintain power and gain more of it. This is all with the goal of a one-world system in which the leader wants undivided worship. We are not free individuals, as the Covid-19 sham has shed light on, and our representatives have long since been bought and paid for. The elites own us, and they are profiting from our misery and pain. When you have the correct worldview, you can see they are agents of Satan. You individually either do the will of God or Satan, it is that simple—so whose camp do you reside in? They do not want you to think independently, so be educated with truth and see them for who they are for they are all sons of Satan.

Check out the scriptural context about Satan taken from **www.gotquestions.org/prince-power-air.html** and you can learn more about who this deceiver and destroyer is and how he operates in the world system he has created.

Physical Conclusions

The following are general suggestions, whether you are in fairly good health and want to be proactive or if you or a loved one are already struggling with health problems.

✓ Find a good integrative medicine doctor. You will most likely have to pay out of pocket but this means these doctors do not have to play by the rules of the system, most can and will do alternative treatments and are free thinkers and willing to listen and try things. They do not treat patients based on dictated protocols from the mainstream system.

✓ Remove all environmental toxins that you can from your home: toxic cleaners, lotions, soaps, deodorant, toothpaste and makeup
  o read the warning label on your toothpaste—two tablespoons will kill you from fluoride
  o find or make your own nontoxic variants of these items
✓ Eat organic and non-GMO foods, especially avoid Bt GMO's and crops treated with Bt (*Bacillus thuringiensis*)

- o Reset gut biome with probiotics, possibly after a mild antibiotic or organic garlic.
- ✓ Stay away from produce with the Apeel label and new mRNA vaccine-laden produce, meat and dairy.
- ✓ Take supplements and make sure they are not synthetic, do not contain titanium, dyes, preservatives, petroleum and other toxins or GMO's
- ✓ Get a reverse osmosis water filter for your drinking water.
- ✓ Use Himalayan or Redmond Real salt, Celtic salt is last choice but no regular table salt.
- ✓ No vaccines
- ✓ Cook your own meals
- ✓ Have mercury dental amalgams (silver fillings) removed with proper safety protocols
- ✓ No processed or boxed foods
- ✓ No fast foods, fried foods, candies or junk foods.
- ✓ Make your own jams, jellies and sweets
- ✓ Start a garden with non-GMO seeds
- ✓ Get chickens, goats and pigs, if you can
- ✓ Start a neighborhood co-op
- ✓ Use butter and lard. NO vegetable shortening, vegetable oil, canola, etc.
- ✓ Use as minimally processed food products as possible
- ✓ Get organized with your church and community
- ✓ Do not send your kids off to daycare and public school every day; it is your job to teach them, not the government's
- ✓ Can and preserve foods or freeze dry if you can afford a machine
- ✓ Most of all, do your homework, study, examine all things and take charge

And the most important of all is to seek for the salvation of your soul, as none of this will matter when you die as you will be instantly standing before God. "And do not be afraid of those who kill the body but are unable to kill the soul; but rather fear Him who is able to destroy both soul and body in hell." Matthew 10:28

Treatment For Metal Toxicity: Chelation Therapy

This will be beneficial for autism, Parkinson's Disease, multiple sclerosis, amyotrophic lateral sclerosis, rheumatoid arthritis, schizophrenia, allergies, endocrine diseases such as hypothyroidism, hyperthyroidism, Hashimoto's Thyroiditis, hyper-parathyroidism, fibromyalgia, most likely everything listing on the back of this book and much more.

Testing

Mercury is cumulative so it is hard to detect because the body stores will not reflect what is tested in urine, blood or hair. The actual body load of these toxins is not accurately represented when you do testing, but testing is essential to see the baseline and to compare what is excreted during chelation. For example, I did a random Urine, twenty-four hour toxic metals urine and a toxic metals hair test from Doctors Data through Directlabs.com. I did a pre- and post-DMSA chelation test of each. Where this testing really helps is showing excretion rates, as well as hidden toxins. In my situation, my pre-chelation amounts of barium and uranium were zero but after a few rounds of chelation they were into the mid-dangerous range. This data also showed it was moving virtually all of the toxic metals on the chart, with the exception of two that I was not exposed to. I did a urine test each month during chelation, the tests look for 20 toxins. DMSA/ALA chelated Aluminum, Antimony, Arsenic, Barium, Bismuth, Cadmium, Cesium, Lead, Mercury, Nickel, Palladium, Tellurium, Thallium, Tin, Tungsten, Uranium. I didn't have Beryllium, Gadolinium, or Platinum but I'm guessing they would chelate them as well for those of you who have had contrasting MRI (gadolinium) or Chemo (platinum)

Chelation Process

If you have amalgam fillings start by removing these. If you have the possibility of having an amalgam-packed root canal, remove these as well. It is a good idea to check with a dentist just to make sure you do not have any amalgam fillings. If none of these apply, start at step 3 to begin a proper chelation process.

1) First find a dentist that is SMART certified (check www.iaomt.org) to remove your amalgams. Do not just go to any dentist, many do not talk about mercury for fear of losing their licenses. The biggest risk of exposure is removal and installment of amalgams. You do not want to risk more exposure at this point. Make sure the dentist uses a dental dam, suctions front and back and utilizes supplemental oxygen. Make sure every last bit of mercury is out before you continue to treatment because if any is left it will leech out and make things worse.

2) After the amalgams are out, find an integrative medicine doctor, unless your doctor is on board with treating you with this specific plan. If not, find a specialist who will follow this protocol. The protocol is called "Andrew Cutler Chelation Protocol" and I would highly suggest buying his book called "The Mercury Detoxification Manual".

(Source: noamalgam.com/product/the-mercury-detoxification-manual/)

The website **andy-cutler-chelation.com** has the basics and the following is the basic idea of chelation therapy and is a summary of the process outlined in his book and on the website.

WARNING: Do not attempt Chelation with amalgams, it will cause mercury to leach out.

Wait four (4) days after amalgam removal before starting chelation therapy.

Do not attempt to use ALA (alpha lipoic acid) before amalgams have been removed, and only after three (3) months have passed can you add ALA to your chelation schedule. Start at low dose 12.5mg. Do not use R-ALA.

Only use prescription DMSA or DMPS as chelators. Natural chelators like cilantro, chlorella, glutathione and EDTA have a weak bond and will cause redistribution of metals to the most sensitive places (brain, thyroid, kidneys and adrenals).

Do not do IV chelation as it is way too high of a dose and will cause a massive redistribution event.

I would encourage you to get the book because it has a wealth of knowledge. Read it and read the complete information on the website before making any decisions.

1. URGENT! REMOVE MERCURY AMALGAMS BEFORE STARTING CHELATION!

It is crucial to prioritize the safe removal of any mercury amalgams from your mouth. Refrain from using any chelating substances while you still have these amalgams or any other mercury exposure (vaccines, pharmaceuticals, etc.).

Only commence the oral chelation protocol after ensuring that you no longer have any mercury amalgams in your mouth.

2. MOST IMPORTANT PRECAUTIONS:

Under no circumstances should you take any form of chelator if you still have mercury in your mouth—amalgam fillings, crowns or any other work with amalgams should be removed first—regardless of advice from doctors or dentists. Disregard any such recommendations.

Avoid IV chelation or challenge tests altogether.

Do not use chlorella or cilantro/coriander for chelation purposes.

3. ORAL CHELATION

Oral chelation is a process where chelating agents are taken orally to bind with metals in the body, forming chemical bonds and reducing the reactivity of the metallic ions. This allows for the safe elimination of these metals through urine or feces.

In normal circumstances, our body uses its glutathione reserves to naturally detoxify and remove small amounts of mercury. However, when the body becomes overwhelmed with metal accumulation, this natural process becomes less effective, leading to a toxic burden and interference with physiological processes.

Mercury tends to accumulate in the body over time and is particularly problematic since it does not easily leave the body, especially from brain tissues. Therefore, oral chelation becomes crucial in removing problematic metals that have built up in the body.

Chelated metals are primarily excreted through the kidneys in urine or through the gastrointestinal tract via the biliary network (bile from the liver) and then excreted in stool.

Mercury is a highly toxic metal widely used in various applications, making it essential to chelate it effectively. Chelation therapy is employed to address mercury toxicity, but it also plays a vital role in removing other metals accumulated through daily exposure and, importantly, from the indiscriminate use of metals in dentistry.

True chelators contain two thiol groups, and their effectiveness lies in this characteristic. However, some health practitioners mistakenly recommend chlorella, cysteine, NAC, and glutathione for chelation. These substances are not true chelators in the chemical sense as they lack two or more binding groups (dithiol groups). Consequently, they are ineffective chelators, and instead of safely excreting metals, they can potentially redistribute stored metals, mobilizing them from their storage sites without effectively binding and removing them. This can lead to further complications, similar to stirring up a hornet's nest.

4. WARNING AGAINST CHALLENGE TESTS, ESPECIALLY DMPS CHALLENGE TEST

Health practitioners sometimes use provoked or challenge tests to assess heavy metal levels in the body through urine, but this can be highly dangerous for individuals with mercury toxicity and should be avoided.

The most common challenge test is the DMPS challenge test, where a large amount of DMPS is given through a single-dose IV injection. This causes the body to release previously bound mercury and other metals from storage sites into the bloodstream. If the body cannot handle this sudden toxic load, it may lead to severe long-term consequences, with many people experiencing adverse effects and permanent damage. Dr. Andy Cutler strongly advises against this test and recommends hair elements testing instead.

DMPS is effective for acute metal toxicity, but as a challenge test, it does not provide reliable information. Even if someone decides to undergo the test, the results cannot be considered meaningful since mercury is mobilized and redistributed throughout the body in unpredictable patterns, making scientific comparisons impossible. DMPS does not cross the blood-brain barrier or cell membranes, offering no information about levels in the brain, organs, and cells.

Challenge tests are discouraged as their results lack meaningful information due to the inconsistent mobilization of mercury, leading to highly variable and skewed readings.

Cautionary Note on EDTA Challenge Test

EDTA challenge tests for individuals with mercury toxicity are also not informative for similar reasons as the DMPS challenge test mentioned above. While EDTA is widely used as an IV chelator, it is not effective in chelating mercury and has a stronger affinity for lead and cadmium. If you are mercury toxic, IV EDTA can potentially worsen the condition.

Instead, it is recommended to follow Dr. Andy Cutler's oral chelation program to safely reduce mercury levels. If necessary, IV EDTA can be considered later, but it can also be used orally for greater safety. Previously, EDTA was promoted as beneficial for removing calcium plaques in blood vessels, but current understanding suggests that it primarily removes metals from the vessel lining (epithelial) receptor sites, freeing up these sites to receive more nitric oxide, which was previously blocked by metals.

5. CHELATING AGENTS FOR MERCURY

DETOXIFICATION

DMSA, DMPS and ALA are effective chelating agents recommended in Dr. Andy Cutler's protocol for mercury detoxification. DMSA, DMPS are prescription drugs so find a doctor who supports your chelation therapy or your best option is likely an integrative medicine doctor. If you are having difficulty finding a willing doctor, call your local pharmacy—a compounding pharmacy is best—and ask for doctors in your area that have prescribed DMSA or DMPS. There are some online doctors that may be able to assist, such as Push Health.

Timing and Order for Chelation

After safely removing all mercury amalgams, wait at least four days before starting with DMSA or DMPS. Add ALA three months later, as it can cleanse the brain and organs by crossing the blood-brain barrier. (Start ALA at a low dose as well 12.5mg, and no R-ALA.)

Importance of Proper Chelation

Correct oral chelation is crucial to avoid problems. Follow Andy Cutler's protocols, build doses up slowly and do not rush the process. Chelators should never be taken if there is still mercury in the mouth, and caution should be exercised with supplement usage to prevent complications.

Chelating Schedule with DMSA and ALA

Start with DMSA alone at 12.5mg every 4 hours for three days ON and three days OFF. Gradually increase the dosage and consider adding ALA after several rounds of DMSA alone. Use both DMSA and ALA together, taking them every three hours during the day, including waking up at night. I personally find that chelating continuously (no days off) at a low/tolerable dose was the best for me, as the days off caused a cumulation of metals without DMSA to remove it leaving me with bad redistribution on days 3-4 off.

Duration of Chelation

Chelation can take anywhere from one to five years to complete, depending on the individual's toxicity level and ability to excrete metals.

Note on Chlorella and Cilantro

Chlorella and cilantro are not effective chelators for mercury and should be avoided, as they can mobilize mercury without properly binding and excreting it.

Continuous Chelation

Chelation should continue for an additional six months to a year after improvement is noticed. Some individuals may need to chelate for several years to achieve optimal results.

Slow and Steady Approach

Chelation is a slow process, and increasing dosages too rapidly can lead to complications. Patience is essential to ensure safe and effective detoxification.

6. SIDE EFFECTS AND CHELATION

Side effects during chelation can vary, increasing or decreasing during each round. Delayed side effects often indicate mobilization of mercury, while immediate side effects may indicate sensitivity to the chelator. To ensure safety, always start with low doses (e.g., 12.5mg of ALA, DMSA or DMPS) to test sensitivity and gradually increase.

The Importance of Patience

Avoid rushing chelation, as hurrying can lead to longer-term complications and slower progress. It is essential to adopt a slow approach, as adverse reactions may emerge in subsequent rounds. Take caution and prioritize your well-being throughout the process.

Symptoms and Mercury Toxicity

Chelation symptoms often confirm mercury toxicity, even if

mercury tests do not show it. Once you can tolerate high doses of safe chelators like ALA (e.g., 1200mg per day) without symptoms, it may suggest a reduction in mercury toxicity. However, progressively worsening side effects with low doses might indicate the presence of hidden amalgam in the mouth.

Chelating with Caution

When experiencing severe symptoms during chelation, it indicates excessive movement of mercury. This should be taken seriously, and adherence to the chelation program, along with a slow buildup, is crucial. Rushing the process can lead to long-term damage and side effects, so avoid being too aggressive in your approach.

Dealing with ALA and Mercury Movement

Some people may face issues when adding ALA, as it moves mercury from the brain and organs. In such cases, reducing the ALA dose significantly (e.g., to 3mg) or continuing with DMSA/DMPS for an extended period before reintroducing ALA is advisable. While ALA is vital for mercury detox, it is essential to find a dose you can tolerate if adverse reactions occur.

Alternative Cancer Treatments

If you or a loved one has cancer, there are hundreds of possible remedies. Cancer takes years or even longer to develop so do not immediately buy the "two weeks to live" line and do not let them use fear to control your actions. Take a step back, pray and do some research as you take control of your health. Almost 30% of people who have cancer and do nothing at all to treat the cancer see it go away completely on its own. Before you do cancer doctor's deadly cancer treatments, research some of these possible remedies. There may be one or more that helps you or your loved one.

Legal disclaimer: I am in no way advocating or instructing any persons on these methods; this information is strictly for informational research purposes. Please consult a knowledgeable integrative medicine specialist before attempting any treatment.

1. **21-day water fasting.** Drink plenty of filtered water with an added level teaspoon of Redmond Real salt or Himalayan salt per gallon to replace electrolytes lost. NO tap water or table salt. Take basic supplements from the supplement chapter. You can juice organic wheat juice shots or take a powdered form but make sure it is organic to limit toxins.

2. **Change your body Ph to alkaline.** Cancer and parasites cannot survive in an alkaline environment, so you want your body to be 7.36 ph. Eliminate sugars as cancer thrives on sugars. Avoid meat, especially red meat, during this time. You can get urine or saliva test strips to test your body ph. Cancer thrives in acidic environments and parasitic infections follow this same pattern.

3. **Sweat it out.** To help your body eliminate waste, use a sauna to sweat out toxins from the body's largest organ, your skin. Spend a few minutes in a sauna until you get a nice sweat and then take a cold shower. This will also stimulate your body's immune response. Do not forget to rehydrate with filtered electrolyte water.

4. **Oxygen therapy.** Find an oxygen therapy specialist who specializes in Prof. Manfred von Ardenne's oxygen treatment therapy. Blood is removed, saturated with ionized oxygen then put back into the body.

5. **Vitamin B17 (laetrile).** This comes from some fruit pits such as apricot and bitter almond. Some doctors say it has a nearly 100% cure rate.

6. **Chinese cancer tree, also Chinese happy tree or *Camptotheca acuminata* or Xi Shu.** The cancer-fighting

of properties of this tree were first verified in 1958 by Dr. Monroe E. Wall of the USDA and Jonathon Hartwell of the National Cancer Institute in the United States.

7. **Essiac tea.** The original recipe was made with four ingredients: burdock root, sheep sorrel, slippery elm and Indian (or Turkish) rhubarb root. A similar product known as "Flor Essence" is made with the same ingredients, plus four additional ones: watercress, blessed thistle, red clover and kelp.

8. **Guanabana leaf tea or extract.** Guanabana extract may prevent or even kill cancer cells without attacking healthy cells for those with many of the most common kinds of cancers. May aid in the treatment and prevention of cancer.

9. **Mistletoe.** A semiparasitic plant that is highly-prescribed in Europe as a cancer treatment. It can be injected directly into the tumor and does not have a high incidence of side effects.

10. **High dose Vitamin C.** Intravenous vitamin C given in a high dose over a sustained number off hours has been seen to safely and sufficiently kill cancer cells in clinical trial.

11. **Hydrogen peroxide therapy.** A small amount of hydrogen peroxide added to water and drunk daily for a specified period has shown results in minimizing cancer. (Source: The Only Answer to Cancer by Dr. Leonard

Coldwell)

12. **Baking soda.** Also an excellent anti-fungal, baking soda can be applied topically, orally, anally, intravenously or even by catheter for direct delivery to the cancer location. As tumors are very acidic, the direct dose of sodium bicarbonate changes the pH to weaken tumors and prevent metastasizing.

Sources: healnavigator.com/treatments/baking-soda-and-cancer and ncbi.nlm.nih.gov/pmc/articles/PMC7249593/

13. <u>**Avermectin**</u> **Class anthelmintics.** This class of drugs is the anti-parasitic drugs such as ivermectin, abamectin, doramectin, eprinomectin, moxidectin and selamectin. As discussed in the cancer chapter of this book, many cancers, if not all, are possibly a type of parasitic infestation. Go to Pubmed.gov and search "Ivermectin Cancer" it will bring up numerous medical journals/studies showing the efficacy of avermectin class drugs against cancers of all types.

14. **Benzimidazole Anthelmintics.** This is another class of anti-parasite drugs such as: fenbendazole, albendazole, ciclobendazole, flubendazole, mebendazole, oxfendazole, oxibendazole, triclabendazole and thiabendazole. *Anecdotally, there are claims that Fenbendazole cured a brain tumor in a veterinarian and another man said it cured his terminal, non-operable lung cancer.*

Nutrition and Supplementation

It is helpful to maintain proper nutrition and supplementation with organic, not synthetic, vitamins. Make sure you eat only organic, non-GMO products as much as possible to prevent even more toxins. Do not get any vaccinations and stay clear of any possible heavy metal exposure.

Post-Chemotherapy Treatment

As we have discussed, chemotherapy is a cocktail of mustard gas nerve agents and heavy metals, mostly platinum. You must get these toxins out of your body and brain. You can do chelation therapy outlined in the section "Treatment for Mercury Toxicity (Chelation Therapy)". You may need the addition of another chelator, sodium thiosulphate, to assist in the specific removal of platinum.

Statin-Induced Myalgia & Dementia

It is not known if much can be done after statin drugs do their damage. They strip the body's nerves of myelin, causing severe damage and nerve and cell necrosis.

Personally, I would cease taking statins immediately and consume as much good cholesterol as possible, specifically in the form of eggs to rebuild the nerve structure. Eat as many eggs as possible by cooking softly scrambled or gently fried eggs, mixing scrambled eggs into shakes or eating soft- or hard-boiled eggs. The more eggs the better! Burn units treat patients with 25+ eggs a day in their diets—food for thought!

Supplement with organic, non-synthetic vitamins and minerals, humic/fulvic acid, chicken collagen powder and beef gelatin.

Arthritis - Rheumatism - Bone Pain - Joint Pain. Take daily chelated calcium, glucosamine sulfate and chondroitin sulfate. Take plain beef gelatin and chicken collagen, one level teaspoon of each in a small glass of orange juice 1-3 times daily to facilitate repair and growth.

Heavy metal and toxin binder. Mix equal parts of food grade gum arabic, calcium bentonite, activated charcoal and zeolite into a storage jar. Take one rounded teaspoon of this mixture in a glass of orange juice daily, as needed. Make sure to take this between medication or supplements by 60-120 minutes or longer as this cocktail will absorb them too.

Headaches. Take Magnesium L-Threonate or Magnesium Glycinate in 300-500mg doses.

Sleep aids. Chamomile, Tilia Estrella, Valarian, Melatonin, GABA

Anxiety. Avoid caffeine, stimulants, high amounts of B vitamins, cayenne and sugars. Take Valarian, magnesium glycinate, L-tryptophan and chamomile. Lavender and lavender oil scent can have a calming effect. Meclizine as over-the-counter Dramamine may help as well.

Canker sores. Rub them with pure alum.

L-Arginine. Helps with blood pressure, healing, erectile disfunction, blood flow, preeclampsia, blood sugar and athletic performance.

Basic Supplements: Vitamins & Minerals

Make sure your supplements are not synthetic. Most synthetics end with "-ate" and "-ide". Make sure they are free from additives like titanium dioxide, polysorbate, glycols, dyes, etc. Make sure they absorb well.

Many common illnesses are caused by lack of nutrition. A good book on this is by Dr. Joel Wallach called *Dead Doctors Don't Lie,* I think he has hit the mark on many things in this book but like everything, do your own research. A good reference book for supplements is *Dr. Earl Mindell's Vitamin Bible.* Here are some recommended basic supplements, these are the basics that are missing in our current diet and can help with many illnesses.

- Get a good daily vitamin that is organic, non-GMO
- Essential amino complex
- Omega 3, 6, 9 (tested for heavy metals)
- Probiotic

- Vitamin D3 (Get outside and get some sun safely without sunscreen)
- Quercetin complex
- Citrus bioflavonoid's
- Chelated calcium
- Full spectrum trace minerals
- Fulvic & Humic mineral blend

APPENDIX A

Spiritual resources:

Read the New Testament of the Bible, perhaps start with the book of John.

Recommended Websites:

www.gracechurch.org

www.GTY.org

www.livingwaters.com

www.ligonier.org

www.heartcrymissionary.com

www.justinpeters.org

www.answersingenesis.org

www.biblegateway.com

www.tms.edu/find-a-church/

www.foundersbaptist.org

Recommended Books:

Holy Bible (New King James version, NASB, LSB) start with the New Testament Book of John

Found: God's Peace by John Macarthur

Found: God's Will by John Macarthur

How to Be Free from the Fear of Death by Ray Comfort

Overcoming Fear, Worry and Anxiety by Elyse Fitzpatrick

The Mercury Detoxification Manual by Rebecca Rust Lee &

Andrew Hall Cutler, PhD, PE

Dr. Earl Mindell's Vitamin Bible

Dead Doctors Don't Lie by Dr. Joel D. Wallach & Dr. Ma Lan

The Only Answer to Cancer by Dr. Leonard Coldwell

It's All In Your Head by Dr. Hal A. Huggins

Solving The Puzzle of Mystery Syndromes by Mary Davis

APPENDIX B

Physical Health Resources

<u>Websites to visit</u>:

www.andy-cutler-chelation.com

www.iaomt.org | The International Academy of Oral Medicine & Toxicology

www.bitchute.com | A place for difficult to find video information, like the "Vaxxed" documentary

www.tv.gab.com | A place for difficult-to-find video information and news

www.EWG.org | Environmental Work Group Tap water database, consumer products testing and more

www.drjwallach.com/Scripts/default.asp | Dr. Wallach's website with vitamin & mineral deficiency info

www.drleonardcoldwell.com | Dr. Leonard Coldwell's site (Cancer Info)

www.AVoiceForChoice.org | Vaccine information

www.DirectLabs.com | They sell Heavy metals test kits (hair, urine, stool) along with many other useful tests delivered to your home.

www.fda.gov/regulatory-information/food-and-drug-administration-modernization-act-fdama-1997/mercury-drug-and-biologic-products

www.childrenshealthdefense.org/

www.childrenshealthdefense.org/wp-content/uploads/2016/10/Federal_Register_4-22-98_Thimerosal_not_GRASE_and_misbranded.pdf

www.childrenshealthdefense.org/wp-

content/uploads/2016/10/1982_Federal_Register_Mercury_in_
OTC_products_ANPR.pdf

APPENDIX C:

FDA SYNTHETIC FLAVORING LIST

https://www.accessdata.fda.gov/scripts/cdrh/cfdocs/cfCFR/CFRSearch.cfm?fr=172.515

Acetal; acetaldehyde diethyl acetal.

Acetaldehyde phenethyl propyl acetal.

Acetanisole; 4'-methoxyacetophenone.

Acetophenone; methyl phenyl ketone.

Allyl anthranilate.

Allyl butyrate.

Allyl cinnamate.

Allyl cyclohexaneacetate.

Allyl cyclohexanebutyrate.

Allyl cyclohexanehexanoate.

Allyl cyclohexaneproprionate.

Allyl cyclohexanevalerate.

Allyl disulfide.

Allyl 2-ethylbutyrate.

Allyl hexanoate; allyl caproate.

Allyl [alpha]-ionone; 1-(2,6,6-trimethyl-2-cyclo-hexene-1-yl)-1,6-heptadiene-3-one.

Allyl isothiocyanate; mustard oil.

Allyl isovalerate.

Allyl mercaptan; 2-propene-1-thiol.

Allyl nonanoate.

Allyl octanoate.

Allyl phenoxyacetate.

Allyl phenylacetate.

Allyl propionate.

Allyl sorbate; allyl 2,4-hexadienoate.

Allyl sulfide.

Allyl tiglate; allyl *trans*- 2-methyl-2-butenoate.

Allyl 10-undecenoate.

Ammonium isovalerate.

Ammonium sulfide.

Amyl alcohol; pentyl alcohol.

Amyl butyrate.

[alpha]-Amylcinnamaldehyde.

[alpha]-Amylcinnamaldehyde dimethyl acetal.

[alpha]-Amylcinnamyl acetate.

[alpha]-Amylcinnamyl alcohol.

[alpha]-Amylcinnamyl formate.

[alpha]-Amylcinnamyl isovalerate.

Amyl formate.

Amyl heptanoate.

Amyl hexanoate.

Amyl octanoate.

Anisole; methoxybenzene.

Anisyl acetate.

Anisyl alcohol; *p*- methoxybenzyl alcohol.

Anisyl butyrate

Anisyl formate.

Anisyl phenylacetate.

Anisyl propionate.

Beechwood creosote.

Benzaldehyde dimethyl acetal.

Benzaldehyde glyceryl acetal; 2-phenyl-*m*- dioxan-5-ol.

Benzaldehyde propylene glycol acetal; 4-methyl-2-phenyl-*m*- dioxolane.

Benzenethiol; thiophenol.

Benzoin; 2-hydroxy-2-phenylacetophenone.

Benzyl acetate.

Benzyl acetoacetate.

Benzyl alcohol.

Benzyl benzoate.

Benzyl butyl ether.

Benzyl butyrate.

Benzyl cinnamate.

Benzyl 2,3-dimethylcrotonate; benzyl methyl tiglate.

Benzyl disulfide; dibenzyl disulfide.

Benzyl ethyl ether.

Benzyl formate.

3-Benzyl-4-heptanone; benzyl dipropyl ketone.

Benzyl isobutyrate.

Benzyl isovalerate.

Benzyl mercaptan; [alpha]-toluenethiol.

Benzyl methoxyethyl acetal; acetaldehyde benzyl [beta]-methoxyethyl acetal.

Benzyl phenylacetate.

Benzyl propionate.

Benzyl salicylate.

Birch tar oil.

Borneol; *d*- camphanol.

Bornyl acetate.

Bornyl formate.

Bornyl isovalerate.

Bornyl valerate.

[beta]-Bourbonene; 1,2,3,3a,3b[beta],4,5,6,6a[beta],6b[alpha]-deca-hydro-l[alpha]-isopropyl-3aa-methyl-6-methylene-cyclobuta [1,2:3,4] dicyclopentene.

2-Butanol.

2-Butanone; methyl ethyl ketone.

Butter acids.

Butter esters.

Butyl acetate.

Butyl acetoacetate.

Butyl alcohol; 1-butanol.

Butyl anthranilate.

Butyl butyrate.

Butyl butyryllactate; lactic acid, butyl ester, butyrate.

[alpha]-Butylcinnamaldehyde.

Butyl cinnamate.

Butyl 2-decenoate.

Butyl ethyl malonate.

Butyl formate.

Butyl heptanoate.

Butyl hexanoate.

Butyl *p*- hydroxybenzoate.

Butyl isobutyrate.

Butyl isovalerate.

Butyl lactate.

Butyl laurate.

Butyl levulinate.

Butyl phenylacetate.

Butyl propionate.

Butyl stearate.

Butyl sulfide.

Butyl 10-undecenoate.

Butyl valerate.

Butyraldehyde.

Cadinene.

Camphene; 2,2-dimethyl-3-methylenenorbornane.

d- Camphor.

Carvacrol; 2-*p-* cymenol.

Carvacryl ethyl ether; 2-ethoxy-*p-* cymene.

Carveol; *p-* mentha-6,8-dien-2-ol.

4-Carvomenthenol; 1-*p-* menthen-4-ol; 4-terpinenol.

cis Carvone oxide; 1,6-epoxy-*p-* menth-8-en-2-one.

Carvyl acetate.

Carvyl propionate.

[beta]-Caryophyllene.

Caryophyllene alcohol.

Caryophyllene alcohol acetate.

[beta]-Caryophyllene oxide; 4-12,12-trimethyl-9-methylene-5-oxatricylo [8.2.0.0 ^{46}] dodecane.

Cedarwood oil alcohols.

Cedarwood oil terpenes.

1,4-Cineole.

Cinnamaldehyde ethylene glycol acetal.

Cinnamic acid.

Cinnamyl acetate.

Cinnamyl alcohol; 3-phenyl-2-propen-1-ol.

Cinnamyl benzoate.

Cinnamyl butyrate.

Cinnamyl cinnamate.

Cinnamyl formate.

Cinnamyl isobutyrate.

Cinnamyl isovalerate.

Cinnamyl phenylacetate.

Cinnamyl propionate.

Citral diethyl acetal; 3,7-dimethyl-2,6-octadienal diethyl acetal.

Citral dimethyl acetal; 3,7-dimethyl-2,6-octadienal dimethyl acetal.

Citral propylene glycol acetal.

Citronellal; 3,7-dimethyl-6-octenal; rhodinal.

Citronellol; 3,7-dimethyl-6-octen-1-ol; *d-* citronellol.

Citronelloxyacetaldehyde.

Citronellyl acetate.

Citronellyl butyrate.

Citronellyl formate.

Citronellyl isobutyrate.

Citronellyl phenylacetate.

Citronellyl propionate.

Citronellyl valerate.

p- Cresol.

Cuminaldehyde; cuminal; *p-* isopropyl benzaldehyde.

Cyclohexaneacetic acid.

Cyclohexaneethyl acetate.

Cyclohexyl acetate.

Cyclohexyl anthranilate.

Cyclohexyl butyrate.

Cyclohexyl cinnamate.

Cyclohexyl formate.

Cyclohexyl isovalerate.

Cyclohexyl propionate.

p- Cymene.

Î³-Decalactone; 4-hydroxy-decanoic acid, Î³-lactone.

Î³-Decalactone; 5-hydroxy-decanoic acid, Î´-lactone.

Decanal dimethyl acetal.

1-Decanol; decylic alcohol.

2-Decenal.

3-Decen-2-one; heptylidene acetone.

Decyl actate.

Decyl butyrate.

Decyl propionate.

Dibenzyl ether.

4,4-Dibutyl-Î³-butyrolactone; 4,4-dibutyl-4-hydroxy-butyric acid, Î³-lactone.

Dibutyl sebacate.

Diethyl malate.

Diethyl malonate; ethyl malonate.

Diethyl sebacate.

Diethyl succinate.

Diethyl tartrate.

2,5-Diethyltetrahydrofuran.

Dihydrocarveol; 8-*p*- menthen-2-ol; 6-methyl-3-isopropenylcyclohexanol.

Dihydrocarvone.

Dihydrocarvyl acetate.

m- Dimethoxybenzene.

p- Dimethoxybenzene; dimethyl hydroquinone.

2,4-Dimethylacetophenone.

[alpha],[alpha]-Dimethylbenzyl isobutyrate; phenyldimethylcarbinyl isobutyrate.

2,6-Dimethyl-5-heptenal.

2,6-Dimethyl octanal; isodecylaldehyde.

3,7-Dimethyl-1-octanol; tetrahydrogeraniol.

[alpha],[alpha]-Dimethylphenethyl acetate; benzylpropyl acetate; benzyldimethylcarbinyl acetate.

[alpha],[alpha]-Dimethylphenethyl alcohol; dimethylbenzyl carbinol.

[alpha],[alpha]-Dimethylphenethyl butyrate; benzyldimethylcarbinyl butyrate.

[alpha],[alpha]-Dimethylphenethyl formate; benzyldimethylcarbinyl formate.

Dimethyl succinate.

1,3-Diphenyl-2-propanone; dibenzyl ketone.

delta-Dodecalactone; 5-hydroxydodecanoic acid, deltalactone.

Î³-Dodecalactone; 4-hydroxydodecanoic acid Î³-lactone.

2-Dodecenal.

Estragole.

Ï쳅-Ethoxybenzaldehyde.

Ethyl acetoacetate.

Ethyl 2-acetyl-3-phenylpropionate; ethylbenzyl acetoacetate.

Ethyl aconitate, mixed esters.

Ethyl Ï쳅-anisate.

Ethyl anthranilate.

Ethyl benzoate.

Ethyl benzoylacetate.

[alpha]-Ethylbenzyl butyrate; [alpha]-phenylpropyl butyrate.

Ethyl brassylate; tridecanedioic acid cyclic ethylene glycol diester; cyclo 1,13-ethyl-enedioxytridecan-1,13-dione.

2-Ethylbutyl acetate.

2-Ethylbutyraldehyde.

2-Ethylbutyric acid.

Ethyl cinnamate.

Ethyl crotonate; *trans*- 2-butenoic acid ethylester.

Ethyl cyclohexanepropionate.

Ethyl decanoate.

2-Ethylfuran.

Ethyl 2-furanpropionate.

4-Ethylguaiacol; 4-ethyl-2-methoxyphenol.

Ethyl heptanoate.

2-Ethyl-2-heptenal; 2-ethyl-3-butylacrolein.

Ethyl hexanoate.

Ethyl isobutyrate.

Ethyl isovalerate.

Ethyl lactate.

Ethyl laurate.

Ethyl levulinate.

Ethyl maltol; 2-ethyl-3-hydroxy-4H-pyran-4-one.

Ethyl 2-methylbutyrate.

Ethyl myristate.

Ethyl nitrite.

Ethyl nonanoate.

Ethyl 2-nonynoate; ethyl octyne carbonate.

Ethyl octanoate.

Ethyl oleate.

Ethyl phenylacetate.

Ethyl 4-phenylbutyrate.

Ethyl 3-phenylglycidate.

Ethyl 3-phenylpropionate; ethyl hydrocinnamate.

Ethyl propionate.

Ethyl pyruvate.

Ethyl salicylate.

Ethyl sorbate; ethyl 2,4-hexadienoate.

Ethyl tiglate; ethyl *trans*- 2-methyl-2-butenoate.

Ethyl undecanoate.

Ethyl 10-undecenoate.

Ethyl valerate.

Eucalyptol; 1,8-epoxy-*p*- menthane; cineole.

Eugenyl acetate.

Eugenyl benzoate.

Eugenyl formate.

Farnesol; 3,7,11-trimethyl-2,6,10-dodecatrien-1-ol.

d- Fenchone; *d*- 1,3,3-trimethyl-2-norbornanone.

Fenchyl alcohol; 1,3,3-trimethyl-2-norbornanol.

Formic acid

(2-Furyl)-2-propanone; furyl acetone.

1-Furyl-2-propanone; furyl acetone.

Fusel oil, refined (mixed amyl alcohols).

Geranyl acetoacetate; *trans*- 3,7-dimethyl-2, 6-octadien-1-yl acetoacetate.

Geranyl acetone; 6,10-dimethyl-5,9-undecadien-2-one.

Geranyl benzoate.

Geranyl butyrate.

Geranyl formate.

Geranyl hexanoate

Geranyl isobutyrate.

Geranyl isovalerate.

Geranyl phenylacetate.

Geranyl propionate.

Glucose pentaacetate.

Guaiacol; Î¼-methoxyphenol.

Guaiacyl acetate; Î¼-methoxyphenyl acetate.

Guaiacyl phenylacetate.

Guaiene; 1,4-dimethyl-7-isopropenyl-[delta]9,10-octahydroazulene.

Guaiol acetate; 1,4-dimethyl-7-([alpha]-hydroxy-isopropyl)-Î´9,10-octahydroazulene acetate.

Î³-Heptalactone; 4-hydroxyheptanoic acid, Î³-lactone.

Heptanal; enanthaldehyde.

Heptanal dimethyl acetal.

Heptanal 1,2-glyceryl acetal.

2,3-Heptanedione; acetyl valeryl.

3-Heptanol.

2-Heptanone; methyl amyl ketone.

3-Heptanone; ethyl butyl ketone.

4-Heptanone; dipropyl ketone.

cis- 4-Heptenal; *cis*- 4-hepten-1-al.

Heptyl acetate.

Heptyl alcohol; enanthic alcohol.

Heptyl butyrate.

Heptyl cinnamate.

Heptyl formate.

Heptyl isobutyrate.

Heptyl octanoate.

1-Hexadecanol; cetyl alcohol.

Ï?-6-Hexadecenlactone; 16-hydroxy-6-hexadecenoic acid, Ï?-lactone; ambrettolide.

Î³-Hexalactone; 4-hydroxyhexanoic acid, Î³-lactone; tonkalide.

Hexanal; caproic aldehyde.

2,3-Hexanedione; acetyl butyryl.

Hexanoic acid; caproic acid.

2-Hexenal.

2-Hexen-1-ol.

3-Hexen-1-ol; leaf alcohol.

2-Hexen-1-yl acetate.

3-Hexenyl isovalerate.

3-Hexenyl 2-methylbutyrate.

3-Hexenyl phenylacetate; *cis-* 3-hexenyl phenylacetate.

Hexyl acetate.

2-Hexyl-4-acetoxytetrahydrofuran.

Hexyl alcohol.

Hexyl butyrate.

[alpha]-Hexylcinnamaldehyde.

Hexyl formate.

Hexyl hexanoate.

2-Hexylidene cyclopentanone.

Hexyl isovalerate.

Hexyl 2-methylbutyrate.

Hexyl octanoate.

Hexyl phenylacetate; *n-* hexyl phenylacetate.

Hexyl propionate.

Hydroxycitronellal; 3,7-dimethyl-7-hydroxy-octanal.

Hydroxycitronellal diethyl acetal.

Hydroxycitronellal dimethyl acetal.

Hydroxycitronellol; 3,7-dimethyl-1,7-octanediol.

N- (4-Hydroxy-3-methoxybenzyl)-nonanamide; pelargonyl vanillylamide.

5-Hydroxy-4-octanone; butyroin.

4-(*p-* Hydroxyphenyl)-2-butanone; *p-* hydroxybenzyl acetone.

Indole.

[alpha]-Ionone; 4-(2,6,6-trimethyl-2-cyclohexen-1-yl)-3-buten-2-one.

[beta]-Ionone; 4-(2,6,6-trimethyl-1-cyclohexen-1-yl)-3-buten-2-one.

[alpha]-Irone; 4-(2,5,6,6-tetramethyl-2-cyclohexene-1-yl)-3-buten-2-one; 6-methylionone.

Isoamyl acetate.

Isoamyl acetoacetate.

Isoamyl alcohol; isopentyl alcohol; 3-methyl-1-butanol.

Isoamyl benzoate.

Isoamyl butyrate.

Isoamyl cinnamate.

Isoamyl formate.

Isoamyl 2-furanbutyrate; [alpha]-isoamyl furfurylpropionate.

Isoamyl 2-furanpropionate; [alpha]-isoamyl furfurylacetate.

Isoamyl hexanoate.

Isoamyl isobutyrate.

Isoamyl isovalerate.

Isoamyl laurate.

Isoamyl-2-methylbutyrate; isopentyl-2-methylbutyrate.

Isoamyl nonanoate.

Isoamyl octanoate.

Isoamyl phenylacetate.

Isoamyl propionate.

Isoamyl pyruvate.

Isoamyl salicylate.

Isoborneol.

Isobornyl acetate.

Isobornyl formate.

Isobornyl isovalerate.

Isobornyl propionate.

Isobutyl acetate.

Isobutyl acetoacetate.

Isobutyl alcohol.

Isobutyl angelate; isobutyl *cis*- 2-methyl-2-butenoate.

Isobutyl anthranilate.

Isobutyl benzoate.

Isobutyl butyrate.

Isobutyl cinnamate.

Isobutyl formate.

Isobutyl 2-furanpropionate.

Isobutyl heptanoate.

Isobutyl hexanoate.

Isobutyl isobutyrate.

[alpha]-Isobutylphenethyl alcohol; isobutyl benzyl carbinol; 4-methyl-1-phenyl-2-pentanol.

Isobutyl phenylacetate.

Isobutyl propionate.

Isobutyl salicylate.

2-Isobutylthiazole.

Isobutyraldehyde.

Isobutyric acid.

Isoeugenol; 2-methoxy-4-propenylphenol.

Isoeugenyl acetate.

Isoeugenyl benzyl ether; benzyl isoeugenol.

Isoeugenyl ethyl ether; 2-ethoxy-5-propenyl-anisole; ethyl isoeugenol.

Isoeugenyl formate.

Isoeugenyl methyl ether; 4-propenylveratrole; methyl isoeugenol.

Isoeugenyl phenylacetate.

Isojasmone; mixture of 2-hexylidenecyclopentanone and 2-hexyl-2-cyclopenten-1-one.

[alpha]-Isomethylionone; 4-(2,6,6-trimethyl-2-cyclohexen-1-yl)-3-methyl-3-buten-2-one; methyl Î³-ionone.

Isopropyl acetate.

ϊ첼-Isopropylacetophenone.

Isopropyl alcohol; isopropanol.

Isopropyl benzoate.

ϊ첼-Isopropylbenzyl alcohol; cuminic alcohol; ϊ첼-cymen-7-ol.

Isopropyl butyrate.

Isopropyl cinnamate.

Isopropyl formate.

Isopropyl hexanoate.

Isopropyl isobutyrate.

Isopropyl isovalerate.

ϊ첼-Isopropylphenylacetaldehyde; ϊ첼-cymen-7-carboxaldehyde.

Isopropyl phenylacetate.

3-(Ϊ챌-Isopropylphenyl)-propionaldehyde; Ϊ챌-isopropylhydrocinnamaldehyde; cuminyl acetaldehyde.

Isopropyl propionate.

Isopulegol; p- menth-8-en-3-ol.

Isopulegone; p- menth-8-en-3-one.

Isopulegyl acetate.

Isoquinoline.

Isovaleric acid.

cis- Jasmone; 3-methyl-2-(2-pentenyl)-2-cyclopenten-1-one.

Lauric aldehyde; dodecanal.

Lauryl acetate.

Lauryl alcohol; 1-dodecanol.

Lepidine; 4-methylquinoline.

Levulinic acid.

Linalool oxide; cis- and trans- 2-vinyl-2-methyl-5-(1'-hydroxy-1'-methylethyl) tetrahydrofuran.

Linalyl anthranilate; 3,7-dimethyl-1,6-octadien-3-yl anthranilate.

Linalyl benzoate.

Linalyl butyrate.

Linalyl cinnamate.

Linalyl formate.

Linalyl hexanoate.

Linalyl isobutyrate.

Linalyl isovalerate.

Linalyl octanoate.

Linalyl propionate.

Maltol; 3-hydroxy-2-methyl-4H-pyran-4-one.

Menthadienol; p- mentha-1,8(10)-dien-9-ol.

p- Mentha-1,8-dien-7-ol; perillyl alcohol.

Menthadienyl acetate; *p*- mentha-1,8(10)-dien-9-yl acetate.

p- Menth-3-en-1-ol.

1-*p*- Menthen--9-yl acetate; *p*- menth-1-en-9-yl acetate.

Menthol; 2-isopropyl-5-methylcyclohexanol.

Menthone; *p* -menthan-3-one.

Menthyl acetate; *p*- menth-3-yl acetate.

Menthyl isovalerate; *p*- menth-3-yl isovalerate.

o- Methoxybenzaldehyde.

p- Methoxybenzaldehyde; *p*- anisaldehyde.

o- Methoxycinnamaldehyde.

2-Methoxy-4-methylphenol; 4-methylguaiacol; 2-methoxy-*p*- cresol.

4-(*p*- Methoxyphenyl)-2-butanone; anisyl acetone.

1-(4-Methoxyphenyl)-4-methyl-1-penten-3-one; methoxystyryl isopropyl ketone.

1-(*p*- Methoxyphenyl)-1-penten-3-one; [alpha]-methylanisylidene acetone; ethone.

1-(*p*- Methoxyphenyl)-2-propanone; anisylmethyl ketone; anisic ketone.

2-Methoxy-4-vinylphenol; *p*- vinylguaiacol.

Methyl acetate.

4'-Methylacetophenone; *p*- methylacetophenone; methyl *p*- tolyl ketone.

2-Methylallyl butyrate; 2-methyl-2-propenl-yl butyrate.

Methyl anisate.

o- Methylanisole; *o*- cresyl methyl ether.

p- Methylanisole; *p*- cresyl methyl ether; *p*- methoxytoluene.

Methyl benzoate.

Methylbenzyl acetate, mixed *o*-,*m*-,*p*-.

[alpha]-Methylbenzyl acetate; styralyl acetate.

[alpha]-Methylbenzyl alcohol; styralyl alcohol.

211

[alpha]-Methylbenzyl butyrate; styralyl butyrate.

[alpha]-Methylbenzyl isobutyrate; styralyl isobutyrate.

[alpha]-Methylbenzyl formate; styralyl formate.

[alpha]-Methylbenzyl propionate; styralyl propionate.

2-Methyl-3-buten-2-ol.

2-Methylbutyl isovalerate.

Methyl *p-tert-* butylphenylacetate.

2-Methylbutyraldehyde; methyl ethyl acetaldehyde.

3-Methylbutyraldehyde; isovaleraldehyde.

Methyl butyrate.

2-Methylbutyric acid.

[alpha]-Methylcinnamaldehyde.

p- Methylcinnamaldehyde.

Methyl cinnamate.

2-Methyl-1,3-cyclohexadiene.

Methylcyclopentenolone; 3-methylcyclopentane-1,2-dione.

Methyl disulfide; dimethyl disulfide.

Methyl ester of rosin, partially hydrogenated (as defined in § 172.615); methyl dihydroabietate.

Methyl heptanoate.

2-Methylheptanoic acid.

6-Methyl-3,5-heptadien-2-one.

Methyl-5-hepten-2-ol.

6-Methyl-5-hepten-2-one.

Methyl hexanoate.

Methyl 2-hexanoate.

Methyl *p-* hydroxybenzoate; methylparaben.

Methyl [alpha]-ionone; 5-(2,6,6-trimethyl-2-cyclohexen-1-yl)-4-penten-3-one.

Methyl [beta]-ionone; 5-(2,6,6-trimethyl-1-cyclohexen-1-yl)-4-penten-3-one.

Methyl [delta]-ionone; 5-(2,6,6-trimethyl-3-cyclohexen-1-yl-)-4-penten-3-one.

Methyl isobutyrate.

2-Methyl-3-(*p*- isopropylphenyl)-propionalde-hyde; [alpha]-methyl-*p*-isopropylhydro- cinnamal- dehyde; cyclamen aldehyde.

Methyl isovalerate.

Methyl laurate.

Methyl mercaptan; methanethiol.

Methyl *o*- methoxybenzoate.

Methyl *N*- methylanthranilate; dimethyl anthranilate.

Methyl 2-methylbutyrate.

Methyl-3-methylthiopropionate.

Methyl 4-methylvalerate.

Methyl myristate.

Methyl [beta]-naphthyl ketone; 2'-acetonaphthone.

Methyl nonanoate.

Methyl 2-nonenoate.

Methyl 2-nonynoate; methyloctyne carbonate.

2-Methyloctanal; methyl hexyl acetaldehyde.

Methyl octanoate.

Methyl 2-octynoate; methyl heptine carbonate.

4-Methyl-2,3-pentanedione; acetyl isobutyryl.

4-Methyl-2-pentanone; methyl isobutyl ketone.

[beta]-Methylphenethyl alcohol; hydratropyl alcohol.

Methyl phenylacetate.

3-Methyl-4-phenyl-3-butene-2-one.

2-Methyl-4-phenyl-2-butyl acetate; dimethylphenylethyl carbinyl acetate.

2-Methyl-4-phenyl-2-butyl isobutyrate; dimethylphenyl ethylcarbinyl isobutyrate.

3-Methyl-2-phenylbutyraldehyde; [alpha]-isopropyl phenylacetaldehyde.

Methyl 4-phenylbutyrate.

4-Methyl-1-phenyl-2-pentanone; benzyl isobutyl ketone.

Methyl 3-phenylpropionate; methyl hydrocinnamate.

Methyl propionate.

3-Methyl-5-propyl-2-cyclohexen-1-one.

Methyl sulfide.

3-Methylthiopropionaldehyde; methional.

2-Methyl-3-tolylpropionaldehyde, mixed *o-, m-, p-.*

2-Methylundecanal; methyl nonyl acetaldehyde.

Methyl 9-undecenoate.

Methyl 2-undecynoate; methyl decyne carbonate.

Methyl valerate.

2-Methylvaleric acid.

Myristaldehyde; tetradecanal.

d- Neomenthol; 2-isopropyl-5-methylcyclohexanol.

Nerol; *cis-* 3,7-dimethyl-2,6-octadien-1-ol.

Nerolidol; 3,7,11-trimethyl-1,6,10-dodecatrien-3-ol.

Neryl acetate.

Neryl butyrate.

Neryl formate.

Neryl isobutyrate.

Neryl isovalerate.

Neryl propionate.

2,6-Nonadien-1-ol.

Î³-Nonalactone; 4-hydroxynonanoic acid, Î³-lactone; aldehyde C-18.

Nonanal; pelargonic aldehyde.

1,3-Nonanediol acetate, mixed esters.

Nonanoic acid; pelargonic acid.

2-Nonanone; methylheptyl ketone.

3-Nonanon-1-yl acetate; 1-hydroxy-3-nonanone acetate.

Nonyl acetate.

Nonyl alcohol; 1-nonanol.

Nonyl octanoate.

Nonyl isovalerate.

Nootkatone; 5,6-dimethyl-8-isopropenyl-bicyclo[4,4,0]-dec-1-en-3-one.

Ocimene; *trans* -[beta]-ocimene; 3,7-dimethyl-1,3,6-octatriene.

Î³-Octalactone; 4-hydroxyoctanoic acid, Î³-lactone.

Octanal; caprylaldehyde.

Octanal dimethyl acetal.

1-Octanol; octyl alcohol.

2-Octanol.

3-Octanol.

2-Octanone; methyl hexyl ketone.

3-Octanone; ethyl amyl ketone.

3-Octanon-1-ol.

1-Octen-3-ol; amyl vinyl carbinol.

1-Octen-3-yl acetate.

Octyl acetate.

3-Octyl acetate.

Octyl butyrate.

Octyl formate.

Octyl heptanoate.

Octyl isobutyrate.

Octyl isovalerate.

Octyl octanoate.

Octyl phenylacetate.

Octyl propionate.

Ï?-Pentadecalactone; 15-hydroxypentadeca-noic acid, Ï?-lactone; pentadecanolide; angelica lactone.

2,3-Pentanedione; acetyl propionyl.

2-Pentanone; methyl propyl ketone.

4-Pentenoic acid.

1-Penten-3-ol.

Perillaldehyde; 4-isopropenyl-1-cyclohexene-1-carboxaldehyde;*p*- mentha-1,8-dien-7-al.

Perillyl acetate; *p*- mentha-1,8-dien-7-yl acetate.

[alpha]-Phellandrene; Ï젤-mentha-1,5-diene.

Phenethyl acetate.

Phenethyl alcohol; [beta]-phenylethyl alcohol.

Phenethyl anthranilate.

Phenethyl benzoate.

Phenethyl butyrate.

Phenethyl cinnamate.

Phenethyl formate.

Phenethyl isobutyrate.

Phenethyl isovalerate.

Phenethyl 2-methylbutyrate.

Phenethyl phenylacetate.

Phenethyl propionate.

Phenethyl salicylate.

Phenethyl senecioate; phenethyl 3,3-dimethylacrylate.

Phenethyl tiglate.

Phenoxyacetic acid.

2-Phenoxyethyl isobutyrate.

Phenylacetaldehyde; [alpha]-toluic aldehyde.

Phenylacetaldehyde 2,3-butylene glycol acetal.

Phenylacetaldehyde dimethyl acetal.

Phenylacetaldehyde glyceryl acetal.

Phenylacetic acid; [alpha]-toluic acid.

4-Phenyl-2-butanol; phenylethyl methyl carbinol.

4-Phenyl-3-buten-2-ol; methyl styryl carbinol.

4-Phenyl-3-buten-2-one.

4-Phenyl-2-butyl acetate; phenylethyl methyl carbinyl acetate.

1-Phenyl-3-methyl-3-pentanol; phenylethyl methyl ethyl carbinol.

1-Phenyl-1-propanol; phenylethyl carbinol.

3-Phenyl-1-propanol; hydrocinnamyl alcohol.

2-Phenylpropionaldehyde; hydratropalde-hyde.

3-Phenylpropionaldehyde; hydrocinnamaldehyde.

2-Phenylpropionalde-hyde dimethyl acetal; hydratropic aldehyde dimethyl acetal.

3-Phenylpropionic acid; hydrocinnamic acid.

3-Phenylpropyl acetate.

2-Phenylpropyl butyrate.

3-Phenylpropyl cinnamate.

3-Phenylpropyl formate.

3-Phenylpropyl hexanoate.

2-Phenylpropyl isobutyrate.

3-Phenylpropyl isobutyrate.

3-Phenylpropyl isovalerate.

3-Phenylpropyl propionate.

2-(3-Phenylpropyl)-tetrahydrofuran.

[alpha]-Pinene; 2-pinene.

[beta]-Pinene; 2(10)-pinene.

Pine tar oil.

Pinocarveol; 2(10)-pinen-3-ol.

Piperidine.

Piperine.

d- Piperitone; *p*- menth-1-en-3-one.

Piperitenone; *p*- mentha-1,4(8)-dien-3-one.

Piperitenone oxide; 1,2-epoxy-*p*- menth-4-(8)-en-3-one.

Piperonyl acetate; heliotropyl acetate.

Piperonyl isobutyrate.

Polylimonene.

Polysorbate 20; polyoxyethylene (20) sorbitan monolaurate.

Polysorbate 60; polyoxyethylene (20) sorbitan monostereate.

Polysorbate 80; polyoxyethylene (20) sorbitan monooleate.

Potassium acetate.

Propenylguaethol; 6-ethoxy-*m*- anol.

Propionaldehyde.

Propyl acetate.

Propyl alcohol; 1-propanol.

p- Propyl anisole; dihydroanethole.

Propyl benzoate.

Propyl butyrate.

Propyl cinnamate.

Propyl disulfide.

Propyl formate.

Propyl 2-furanacrylate.

Propyl heptanoate.

Propyl hexanoate.

Propyl *p*- hydroxybenzoate; propylparaben.

3-Propylidenephthalide.

Propyl isobutyrate.

Propyl isovalerate.

Propyl mercaptan.

[alpha]-Propylphenethyl alcohol.

Propyl phenylacetate.

Propyl propionate.

Pyroligneous acid extract.

Pyruvaldehyde.

Pyruvic acid.

Rhodinol; 3,7-dimethyl-7-octen-1-ol; *l*- citronellol.

Rhodinyl acetate.

Rhodinyl butyrate.

Rhodinyl formate.

Rhodinyl isobutyrate.

Rhodinyl isovalerate.

Rhodinyl phenylacetate.

Rhodinyl propionate.

Rum ether; ethyl oxyhydrate.

Salicylaldehyde.

Santalol, [alpha] and [beta].

Santalyl acetate.

Santalyl phenylacetate.

Skatole.

Sorbitan monostearate.

Sucrose octaacetate.

[alpha]-Terpinene.

Î³-Terpinene.

[alpha]-Terpineol; *p*- menth-1-en-8-ol.

[beta]-Terpineol.

Terpinolene; *p*- menth-1,4(8)-diene.

Terpinyl acetate.

Terpinyl anthranilate.

Terpinyl butyrate.

Terpinyl cinnamate.

Terpinyl formate.

Terpinyl isobutyrate.

Terpinyl isovalerate.

Terpinyl propionate.

Tetrahydrofurfuryl acetate.

Tetrahydrofurfuryl alcohol.

Tetrahydrofurfuryl butyrate.

Tetrahydrofurfuryl propionate.

Tetrahydro-pseudo-ionone; 6,10-dimethyl-9-undecen-2-one.

Tetrahydrolinalool; 3,7-dimethyloctan-3-ol.

Tetramethyl ethylcyclohexenone; mixture of 5-ethyl-2,3,4,5-tetramethyl-2-cyclohexen-1-one and 5-ethyl-3,4,5,6-tetramethyl-2-cyclohexen-1-one.

2-Thienyl mercaptan; 2-thienylthiol.

Thymol.

Tolualdehyde glyceryl acetal, mixed *o, m, p.*

Tolualdehydes, mixed *o, m, p.*

p- Tolylacetaldehyde.

o- Tolyl acetate; *o*- cresyl acetate.

p- Tolyl acetate; *p*- cresyl acetate.

4-(*p*- Tolyl)-2-butanone; *p*- methylbenzylacetone.

p- Tolyl isobutyrate.

p- Tolyl laurate.

p- Tolyl phenylacetate.

2-(*p*- Tolyl)-propionaldehyde; *p*- methylhydratropic aldehyde.

Tributyl acetylcitrate.

2-Tridecenal.

2,3-Undecadione; acetyl nonyryl.

Î³-Undecalactone; 4-hydroxyundecanoic acid Î³-lactone; peach aldehyde; aldehyde C-14.

Undecenal.

2-Undecanone; methyl nonyl ketone.

9-Undecenal; undecenoic aldehyde.

10-Undecenal.

Undecen-1-ol; undecylenic alcohol.

10-Undecen-1-yl acetate.

Undecyl alcohol.

Valeraldehyde; pentanal.

Valeric acid; pentanoic acid.

Vanillin acetate; acetyl vanillin.

Veratraldehyde.

Verbenol; 2-pinen-4-ol.

Zingerone; 4-(4-hydroxy-3-methoxyphenyl)-2-butanone.

ABOUT THE AUTHOR

Harold Godspeed is an Army veteran, former federal police officer, expert mechanic, father of seven and follower of Jesus Christ. His interests include evangelism, helping others, research and development, gardening, cooking, science experiments, cars and rodents of all kinds. He is a true Renaissance Man. After discovering the root cause of his many health problems, he is passionate about reaching others with the truth of our medical system, food and drug corporations and government coverups so that others can find health and life.

www.ingramcontent.com/pod-product-compliance
Lightning Source LLC
Chambersburg PA
CBHW070105030426

42335CB00016B/2018